IN VITRO FERTILIZATION

IN VITRO FERTILIZATION,

BUILDING POLICY FROM LABORATORIES TO LEGISLATURES

Andrea L. Bonnicksen

COLUMBIA UNIVERSITY PRESS
New York

Library of Congress Cataloging-in-Publication Data

Bonnicksen, Andrea L.
In vitro fertilization: building policy from laboratories to legislatures
p.   cm.
Bibliography: p.
Includes index.
ISBN 0-231-06904-9
1. Fertilization in vitro, Human—Social aspects—United States.
2. Fertilization in vitro, Human—Government policy—United States.
3. Fertilization in vitro, Human—Law and legislation—United States.
I. Title.
RG135.B66   1989   362.1′98178—dc19   88-34620
CIP

Columbia University Press
New York   Oxford
Copyright © 1989 Columbia University Press
All rights reserved
Printed in the United States of America

Casebound editions of Columbia University Press books are
Smyth-sewn and printed on permanent and durable acid-free paper

c 10 9 8 7 6 5 4 3

To my sister Linda

Contents

Acknowledgments		ix
1.	Beginning an Era of Choice	1
2.	Tracking the Symbols of In Vitro Fertilization	11
3.	The Responsible Physician	25
4.	The Responsible Patient	51
5.	A Responsible Government	75
6.	A Responsible Public	117
7.	Looking to the Future	137
	Appendix: The IVF Technique	147
	Notes	153
	Bibliography	177
	Index	191

Acknowledgments

The list grew long very quickly of people who shared with me their time and thoughts about in vitro fertilization. I am especially indebted to Dr. Anne Colston Wentz of Vanderbilt University Medical Center, Dr. Jan Friberg of Mount Sinai Hospital Medical Center, and Dr. Edward Marut of Michael Reese Hospital, who opened their doors to my earliest inquiries about alternative conception. I am also grateful to physicians and scientists at the University of Washington Hospital, Swedish Hospital Medical Center, Yale University School of Medicine, University of Texas Medical Branch, University of Texas Health Sciences Center, University of Virginia Medical Center, Jones Institute for Reproductive Medicine, and Oregon Health Science University School of Medicine, among others, for their graciousness in responding to my questions.

Nurse coordinators and other IVF team members at many of these centers drew my attention to IVF from the point of view of the patient. I wish especially to thank Catherine Garner, Filomena Nero, Donna Creech, and Pattei Lazear. The patients themselves, with their stories of infertility and the hope offered by IVF, educated me about the human side of IVF and fed curiosity about the reasons for the many contradictions between the private world of IVF and the public reaction to it.

I am very thankful to the American Philosophical Society and the National Endowment for the Humanities for awarding grants that made possible a two-month stay at the Hastings Center as a Visiting Scholar. At the Hastings Center I learned the value of examining and coaxing ideas at leisure in the expectation that they would yield continually unfolding meanings. I also came to appreciate the solemnity with which caring persons can ask of a biomedical technique, "Is this good?"

The American Political Science Association funded a research trip to Texas that allowed me to interview staff members at hospitals in Galveston and Houston and to spend several days at the Institute for the Medical Humanities in Galveston, where computerized library searches and discussions with faculty members helped me clarify fledgling ideas. The Council for Faculty Research at Eastern Illinois University provided financial support for travel, telephone calls, and a mail survey to the directors of the nation's IVF centers. I wish to thank these organizations.

Other help and insight came from James Childress, William Winslade, John C. Fletcher, Patricia A. King, Walter Harrelson, Richard M. Zaner, and Bruce Jennings. Special thanks go to Juliana Helmke, who read early drafts of papers on IVF; Kay Noeth-Sharp and Declan Hall, who helped with library searches; and Bud May of the Office of Research and Grants, who took extra steps to help develop strategy to finance parts of my research. Kate Wittenberg of Columbia University Press has been a consistently patient and encouraging editor. She had much to do with getting this manuscript off the ground and keeping it there. For steadfast and valued moral encouragement, I give special thanks to Ed Brazil of Eastern Illinois University.

Unattributed quotations in the pages below are from some of the dozens of people who openly talked about IVF. Not all will agree with my conclusions. Their readiness to observe and ponder bears comforting witness to the ability of persons in a pluralistic society to manage the challenges posed by reproductive technologies in the decades to come.

IN VITRO FERTILIZATION

All things human have two aspects, much as the Silenes of Alcibiades, who had two utterly opposed faces; and thus, what at first looked like death, when closely observed was life.

Erasmus, *In Praise of Folly*

CHAPTER ONE

Beginning an Era of Choice

Four years ago I talked with Maria, a woman who unsuccessfully tried in vitro fertilization (IVF) and whom I was interviewing as part of my research on reproductive technologies. "The best part is hope," she said, "and the sad part is packing your car and going home."

Speaking with a soft southern accent, Maria told me that she had been trying to have a baby for seven years. Two IUDs had been imbedded in her uterus and had left her with adhesions that blocked her fallopian tubes. The doctor who had put in and taken out each IUD had never mentioned that Maria would be infertile from the experience. After four unsuccessful surgeries to clear her fallopian tubes, she signed up for IVF.

"I'm not a lucky person," she said of her decision to try IVF. "But I thought this time, 'I'm going to beat the odds.' We knew that this was it. There is only so much surgery your body can tolerate and this was it." For Maria, the attempt was "it" in the final sense. Her single attempt at IVF failed in its early stages. She, who had been among the first to try the IUD and was now among the first to try IVF, did not gain from the promise of either technique.

Maria's story touched me and I thought of it in my library research when I came across talk of test-tube babies, genetic engineering, white-coated scientists, Nazism, artificial wombs, and repeated references to the ethical and moral dilemmas of the new reproductive technologies. In vitro fertilization, it seemed, wore two faces. To some observers, it brought with it the capacity to depersonalize and carry society down a slope of increasingly negative applications. To others, it was a simple medical technique offering hope to people in need. At times the pictures painted were so contradictory that it was hard to believe the observers were talking about the same technique.

In an effort to understand more about the riddle of IVF, I began visiting IVF centers, ethics institutes, and libraries where I secured over six hundred sources ranging from journal, magazine, and newspaper articles to books written by persons in a variety of fields. Throughout, I learned to respect the buoyancy of the topic of IVF. What seemed sinister to one person seemed natural to another. What was a harbinger of evil consequences to some was a window of opportunity for others. Even the image of the "test-tube baby" drew fundamentally different reactions. In a 1972 edition of the *Saturday Review* a drawing in an article on IVF pictured an infant suspended forlornly in a giant test tube—the ultimate depersonalized and dehumanized enterprise.[1] In contrast, brightly painted posters hang on the doors of some IVF clinics, showing rosy-cheeked babies diving into a swimming pool shaped like a giant test tube—the ultimate cheerful pursuit.

Physicians and nurse coordinators at IVF centers welcomed me, a stranger, with warmth and openness. In response to my requests, they contacted patients who in turn called me to talk about their experiences. Most, like Maria, had not gotten pregnant with IVF. Still, they were loyal supporters of IVF, happy they had tried and committed to the hope it offered. Even those who complained about their experiences quickly said, "try it," when asked what advice they would give to other women considering signing up for IVF.

At one center I attended "egg classes," watched ultrasound monitoring, talked to couples in waiting rooms, and sat in on a staff meeting. At another, I witnessed egg retrieval surgeries and took notes that showed a continued curiosity about IVF's conflicting messages. A slick, controlling procedure by blank-faced laboratory technicians this was not. Instead, amid the competence of the physicians, I saw signs of something unexpected—homeliness. One patient walked into the surgical chamber carrying her street clothes in a plastic bag. During the surgery, the test tubes holding the contents of her now-drained follicules were propped in a bed of heated marbles (an incubator) like a basket of flowers. A handmade sign on the box read "egg warmer." An assistant checked off on a bulletin board with a Magic Marker each follicle as it was drained and he read a book while waiting to make the next entry. Afterwards, in the cramped laboratory room where the eggs were prepared for fertilization, I was scooted out of the room when the woman's husband was brought

2

in and given a paper cup for producing his semen. As if entering a sanctuary, he removed his baseball cap before going into the laboratory.

At one hospital I watched two embryo transfers, which are the office procedures in which embryos are inserted into the prospective mother. I had read charges of IVF as a dehumanizing procedure. At first glance it seemed to be true. The room, rigorously antiseptic, was cold and gleaming. Then the woman was rolled in on a stretcher with her husband walking alongside holding her hand and carrying a Louis d'Amour paperback. The physician, nurse, and embryologist walked in cracking jokes about "two eggs, over easy" and "sunnyside up." We all watched the ultrasound screen as the doctor inserted the catheter into the woman and the embryos were released from the hollow tube with a barely visible woosh. "Go on little fellow, do your stuff." "Twins." "No, triplets." "Please, one will do fine." At the end, a nurse brought in a muffin with a candle. It was the doctor's birthday. He blew out the candle and made no secret of his wish. If he had his way a baby would be conceived that day.

The articles arriving at the inter-library loan desk carried a different message and I tried to look beneath the surface to find cracks in the seams of IVF. Physicians and patients to whom I talked also pointed part of the way. There were "charlatans" out there, one andrologist said, and patients were being "ripped off" by clinics that admitted anyone who walked through their doors. As for future applications, certainly, an endocrinologist thought, there was a possibility of embryo trafficking: "You never know what a physician is going to do."

I accommodated my research to the unsettling pace of technological change. The addition of embryo freezing took me on a new round of interviews and photocopying of articles written by worried authors that underscored the same schizophrenic quality about reactions to IVF that I had earlier noted. Freezing would raise "extremely difficult," "thorny," "enormously complex," and even "nightmarish" ethical and legal dilemmas, writers warned. Directors of IVF clinics had a different prediction, however: freezing was a cutting edge service about which they and their patients were excited. Freezing, they said, furthered the practitioner's ability to store and study human embryos in order to understand human reproduction, learn about contraception, prevent genetic defects, and examine the course of adult diseases. By this time I was hearing and reading about how IVF was a "window" to help infertile couples . . . and the rest of society too. From the early slippery slope metaphor, in which people predicted IVF would take us *down* a slope of accelerating negative consequences, people now predicted that IVF would take us *up* to a future of accelerating wonderful consequences for the understanding of adult disease, contraception, and the prevention of genetic defects. Health and vitality were in the wind. In vitro fertilization had a new hat to wear: that of savior.

During all this, one colleague kept asking when I was going to get the book published: "Things are changing so fast, you've got to get it out." By this time I had figured out that the book would not be dated because the techniques might change at a furious pace but the underlying questions do not. There is unfinished business here that will not rest; on the contrary, it will become more palpable as techniques change. We have upon our backs the weight of unresolved polarity about basic IVF and we have failed to take account of the areas of consensus that lie hidden beneath the headlines and flamboyant symbols. Our understanding about how we have reacted to IVF is stubbornly incomplete.

We have courted diverse images of IVF with equal passion (IVF as monster, savior, and neutral medical technique), lived with a federal government that has sat out the issue because it is a "hot potato," and tried to fathom diametrically opposed viewpoints as to IVF's inherent goodness for society. It is enticing to forge ahead and to embrace new techniques of freezing, tissue donation, and genetic manipulation in a flurry of choice. Yet doing so is not unlike a person marrying and divorcing once, then twice, three times, four times, and yet a fifth time without stopping to wonder about the underlying reasons for the dismal record. At some point we need to come to grips with what is already before us and to examine our record. Are we as divided as sometimes appears? Is IVF as dramatic and controversial as some would have us believe? Or is our record of achievement more substantial than we realize?

Questions remain that we as a society must face about integrating IVF and its variations into our world and deciding how to respond to these developments. Infertility treatment is a newly respectable area of medicine, which gained credibility with the birth of the first "test-tube baby" in 1978. Medicine is part of our culture. What kind of interaction do we expect between doctor and patient in the field of new conceptions? How do we respond to a technique that is a medical choice but not a medical necessity? Do we bring it into the medical world happily?

Despite a history of limited federal involvement in IVF, legislators are now moving to regulate IVF and help couples secure access to reproductive technologies. How much involvement do we want from the government in the administration of the technologies? Is IVF primarily a private or public matter? Do we want to invite increased government oversight?

Or do we prefer to leave the monitoring to the private sector? Do we want to place public resources behind these new techniques?

Further, what does our reaction to IVF tell us about our own social values? Why should we care about these techniques? Why have we responded with such a strange mixture of attraction and repulsion? What does our language tell us about our values? What does it mean to talk about "test-tube babies" and "miracle" babies and "desperate" patients? Why do we both deify and satanize a technique that unites microscopic eggs and sperm in a Pyrex petri dish?

Above all, what is our role as citizens in the oversight and management of new reproductive techniques? In vitro fertilization and its variations offer choice, if not to us, then to our children. A daughter born today will have a wealth of choice about when and how to conceive her own children. Already women have donated eggs to their anovulatory sisters, a woman has given birth to her daughter's genetic triplets, and scientists are talking of cutting off portions of embryos to study for chromosomal abnormalities. Does the prospect of our daughters and sons storing embryos at age twenty-one for delayed childbearing sound desirable? Does the ability to analyze embryos destined to be our grandchildren and great-grandchildren seem tantalizing or disconcerting?

The history of the technique of IVF roughly falls into three time periods of exploration, consolidation, and expansion. The years of exploration reached their peak from 1969 to 1978, when the first baby was born after having been fertilized externally. From this era came "basic IVF," the fertilization of a wife's fresh ova and a husband's fresh sperm for immediate transfer to the wife's uterus.

The period of consolidation has lasted from 1978 to the present. During this time IVF has become integrated into medical practice so that many physicians talk about it as a first resort, not a last resort for tubal infertility. Around 170 clinics offer IVF across the country and, for the first time, insurance companies are reimbursing couples for part or all of it. During this time IVF has lost its ability to shock.

Contentment with techniques is perhaps anathema to the American growth ethic, and the stage of consolidation has been supplanted by an era of "expanded IVF," starting in about 1984, with the first birth of an infant that had been frozen as an embryo. Expanded IVF overlaps with the era of consolidation and moves us forward at a disconcerting pace. Expanded IVF brings with it the freezing and storage of human sperm, eggs, and embryos; donation of these tissues to other couples; introduction of third and fourth parties as tissue donors; and the study of human embryos for genetic diagnosis.

In these early years of expanded IVF, we can assess our roles as participants and consumers of new conceptions. On the one hand, we can move along a path of largely uncircumspect consumption in which we embrace the new techniques with little societal introspection about them. Here we consume without understanding why, accept techniques without comprehending their purpose, and march forward with a vague sense that we may not want to be marching. New goods and services beckon and we take them because they are there for the offering. Our vision of the future is linear, even though at times tinged with resignation. We speak of the technological imperative ("what can be done will be done") with a curious mixture of optimism and powerlessness. We assume the benefits of research and knowledge and are confident problems in technology can be answered with more technology. If we consume all that expanded IVF has to offer we are exhibiting faith of the sort that has propelled us through the centuries since the European Middle Ages.

On the other hand, we can move toward a path of circumspect consumption which involves deliberate efforts to limit technology where doing so appears to fill a greater societal need than embracing the technology. A measure of self-knowledge comes with this approach preceeded by an understanding of for whom and for what progress is thought desirable. To question linear consumption is, however, disconcerting. It is like taking a person who revels in the finely detailed portraits of the Flemish masters into a room of paintings of Picasso, with eyes and noses akimbo. Just as the cubist art form distorts perceptions thought to be truthful renditions of reality, so does the questioning of unlimited technology distort the very assumptions of ourselves as consumers of new techniques.

The following chapters adhere to the belief that we must evaluate priorities and values now, in the early stages of expanded IVF, before advancing further. To move ahead with self-knowledge and self-understanding is to progress; to advance into expanded IVF with the weight of unresolved polarities and with an unclear understanding of ourselves as consumers is to regress. If anything, expanded IVF ought to open reproductive choice (both to say yes and no) rather than close us to determinism. For this we need to understand our responsibilities as individuals faced with the panorama of choice. We need to understand how each of IVF's communities of patients, physicians and scientists, policymakers, and the general public can assume responsibility for circumspect consumption of changing reproductive techniques.

A premise of the following chapters is that the rudiments of a consensus exist but are hidden behind sensationalism and complaints about governmental incompetence. We agree about more values and have made more progress in policymaking than is often recognized. While problems, quandaries, and questions arise, they fall short of crises. From this consensus comes the building blocks of a policy of limited consumption. The policy glass is, by the perspective taken in this book, half-full, not half-empty, but we cannot assume the moment will wait indefinitely. Instead, with expanded IVF, our ability to put limits may diminish as the pulse of technological change fades into our unconscious and untested values.

According to Michael Gregory, "Values are ideas that have become part of a cultural tradition, an established worldview—so much a part that they tend to be transmitted unconsciously from generation to generation."[2] The evolution of values is gradual, delicate, and nearly imperceptible. Alfred North Whitehead once said of the "form of thought" of each historical period, "like the air we breathe, such a form is so translucent, and so pervading, and so seemingly necessary, that only by extreme effort can we become aware of it."[3]

In this book I suggest that we are at a stage where we can still observe the values relating to IVF as they emerge. This stage is already changing, however, as our values become increasingly silent in their formation and as the persons who are influential in our value change—physicians, patients, and scientists—are withdrawing from the vivid public surveillance of IVF's early years. We will need increasingly greater acts of will and effort to be aware of the subtly changing values in our thought that will push us toward indiscriminant consumption.

As we read about our consumption-oriented society, a society in which nearly 250 new products ranging from Squirms (worm-shaped jelly beans) to pens for writing on fingernails are patented each month,[4] it becomes clear that the choices and alternatives offered by expanded IVF are not so very different from other choices in our society. I will illustrate by way of a homely analogy using a microwavable hot-fudge sundae.

Several decades ago, the microwave oven was invented and marketed for use in home kitchens. It was, to set the stage for the analogy, a "basic microwave." But the microwave ran into troubles. It emitted radiation through leaks in the doors and it interfered with another modern invention, the pacemaker. Once these problems were fixed, the microwave was free to be purchased and used at will by consumers. The problem, however, was that consumers could not be counted on to buy the machines; the food did not brown, look nice, or taste good. This prompted

7

a series of steps to turn the microwave into a useful machine. Companies invented turning trays for a more even distribution of cooking; perfected microwavable dishes, tools, and recipes; and refined time settings to make microwave cooking more sophisticated. When that was not enough, companies invented prepackaged microwavable foods and competed for shelf space in frozen food sections of food markets.

Still, families persisted in underutilizing microwaves by using them primarily to boil water and reheat leftovers. How could manufacturers get people to use the appliances to prepare full meals? More was done to make microwave food palatable; today it is not just revolving trays or microwave cake mixes, but the containers that are the object of research. The newest refinements are special plates that allow the crust of pizza or the top of the fish patty to get brown, "microready indicators" to take the guesswork out of microwaving, and, the ultimate, the microwavable sundae, in which the packaging lets the fudge molecules "get excited" while the ice cream molecules, in their bottom cocoon, stay cool.[5]

The microwave has taken on as frenetic an activity as the molecules it is supposed to stir up. Since the basic microwave has come to the market, there has been no logical stopping place for expanded microwavery. By now the needs have been created and the value absorbed: if there is a problem a new technology will resolve it. It is no longer an alternative to go back to ovens. Once the microwave was introduced, it became fixable, improvable, and, stubbornly but finally in the mind of consumers, valuable.

The analogy, of course, can be applied to IVF, with basic IVF akin to the basic microwave and expanded IVF as something that can take on the same self-energizing justification as microready indicators and nonexcitable ice cream molecules. Far be it for persons to call a halt and suggest going back to the old way. The danger lies not in technology itself, but in the subtle value changes that foreclose possibilities once thought perfectly legitimate. Before getting to that stage, we can ask if expansion will improve our society in a definite way. Does expansion increase free choice? Or does it create consumers as victims who respond to created needs, trying ever onward to make that food palatable?

With IVF we are at that juncture. Maria said the failed IVF attempt "was it" but, in the next breath, said:

> "We will go surrogate next. I am not the type of person to give up. We also thought of ovum transfer. My sister is almost my identical twin. She may give us an egg. This is our next thought. We will talk with her this weekend about it."

8

Would Maria be better off knowing there were no more alternatives for biological parenthood? Is she now, four years later, back at an infertility clinic, trying to arrange egg or embryo donation with her sister or a surrogate? How best can we evaluate the goodness of expanded IVF? How best can we respond as responsible citizens to something imperceptibly changing in our societal landscape?

The time to ask these questions is now, while we are still wondering and before the form becomes "translucent and pervading" and more and more difficult to see. The following chapters are united by the message that each IVF community—physicians, patients, policymakers, and the attentive public—has before it ways of calling limits and assuming responsibility for the circumspect consumption of new conceptions.

CHAPTER TWO

Tracking the Symbols of
In Vitro Fertilization

We build our lives around symbols. With symbols we organize, communicate, and define our everyday reality. Symbols weave throughout our world and, after time, take a power of their own. Like money, they elicit emotions and reactions long after the first meaning is lost. They have the ability to "induce actions, feelings, emotions, and beliefs about things which are mere notions."[1]

The medical field has within it symbols of doctors in white coats and dangling stethoscopes who connote healing. Diseases carry powerful symbolic meanings. Tuberculosis, cancer, leprosy, polio, and, more recently, AIDS elicit by their very word an emotional response. With in vitro fertilization, we have attached a wealth of meanings to a technique — the making of the "test-tube baby."

Few medical techniques have attracted as varied a symbolic response as IVF. The first modern indications that scientists were trying to fertilize a human egg externally provoked an at-times cacophonous medley of symbols from an "army of pundits"[2] including journalists, sociologists, theologians, physicians, and at least one Nobel prize winner. That army spoke loudly up to the birth of the first baby from IVF in 1978, after which it has been supplanted, subtly and gradually, by the physicians and scientists who practice IVF. With this changing of the guard has come a new symbolic legacy that justifies IVF and pushes us in the direction of linear consumption of infertility techniques. Our ability to question that consumption begins with an understanding of how and by whom our reality about IVF is defined.

THE BIRTH OF IN VITRO FERTILIZATION

The motivation that led to IVF dates to a long-standing effort to make fertile those who are infertile. Local religions, superstitions, beliefs, and materials have created a legacy of remedies for women and men to drink, eat, rub, and insert. Physicians in the time of Hippocrates advised women to eat "butter in the morning on an empty stomach and [drink] milk from a woman nursing a boy." If she belched, she would conceive. "[I]f not, no." Men were thought to be sterile if they had had an incision above the neck, in which case "semen passes from the head alongside the ears to the spinal cord; however, that passage becomes hardened by the scar that arises from the incision."[3]

The attempt to understand infertility and reproduction has advanced in an uneven rythmn. In the time of Aristotle it was thought that fetuses stayed small but pre-formed within the woman and grew upon their "unshelling." Scientists in the early 1600s anticipated the modern theory of reproduction that women produce eggs and that the embryo grows gradually after sperm and egg unite. A Dutch scientist, Reinier de Graaf, described the process but was wrong in one critical respect: he had seen the ovaries of cattle coagulate when boiled and he thought that the human egg, like a boiled hen's egg, was a white mass filling one ovary.[4]

In 1827 modern discoveries started when scientists identified mammalian ova outside the body. This was followed by an external fertilization of mammalian egg and sperm in 1875 and the viewing of human ova for the first time in the 1930s. In the 1940s one physician paired human ova with sperm in vitro but he did not document a fertilization.[5]

With these discoveries, that which had been a mystery became visible and observable. In a sense, it was a letdown from the myth and legend handed down over the centuries. Where, for example, would a novelist be who had written not of rapture and conjugal bliss but of the spermatozoa's trek up the cervical tract? Were it not for misinformation about conception where would be the amulets, statues, and legends groomed by societies trying to ensure and celebrate fertility? When Landrum Shettles published the first photographs of a cleaving human embryo in the mid 1950s, it looked as if science had handed us an anticlimax.[6] No gargantuan stone phalluses were these. Instead, the photographs in the article "A Morula Stage of Human Ovum Developed In Vitro" presented, in magnified black and white, a cleaving egg that looked like a photocopied reproduction of a mound of caviar. It gave little grist for literary imagination.

On the other hand, to observe human gametes was an astonishing development in light of the primitive theories entertained over the years. One physician wrote, in his introduction to a book picturing fertilizing eggs, that we had taken "a large step in our quest for understanding of the beginnings of human life."[7] In 1969 the first scientifically reported results of in vitro fertilization were published by a British physiologist, Robert Edwards, and a gynecologist, Patrick Steptoe.[8]

To Edwards and Steptoe, the unlocking of the mysteries of human conception was a beauty in itself. Upon their first fertilization, Steptoe said, "A fertilized human egg! . . . I am one of the three or four people in the world who has genuinely seen this phenomenon." Edwards was no less enthralled:

We had a feeling of being greatly privileged to see those human blastocysts.

I knew that instant that we had reached our goal: the early stages of human life were all there in our culture fluids, just as we wanted. . . . and even as I gazed down at those embryos, wondering what to do with them, there was no doubt in my mind that the whole field was now wide open.[9]

How bold were the hopes of these two men and the scores of women who participated in their effort over the next decade to transfer the embryos to women's uteruses in order to achieve a pregnancy. Steptoe looked at the backlog of his infertility patients and thought that his IVF work would give him a "chance indeed to uphold the rights of women and alleviate, as my mother would have wished, some of the wrongs done to them." When Edwards, the father of five daughters, saw a human egg preparing itself for fertilization by its march of chromosomes, he felt positively biblical: "Why, it meant that possibly infertility in some women could be cured. The angel could come to Sarah." For them, IVF symbolized hope, service, knowledge, and, as well, personal gain and scientific achievement. There was nothing troublesome about this technique. On the contrary, wrote Edwards: "I had no doubts about the morals and ethics of our work. I accepted the right of our patients to found their family, to have their own children."[10]

In vitro fertilization was still to show its resilient ability to ensnare imaginations, however. The idea of human reproduction being started in a glass dish enlisted, outside of Edwards' laboratory, an amalgam of

13

concern, shock, excitement, and outrage such as had rarely, if ever, attended a scientific development. It was, said one, *the* event of modern times: "No other recent development in biological engineering has raised as much doubt among the public as that involving experiments in which conception has been carried out, and gestation fostered, in a test tube."[11]

For its part, the popular press picked up the imagery of test-tube babies lingering from the publication in 1932 of Aldous Huxley's *Brave New World*.[12] The *New York Times* announced that "Life Is Created in a Test Tube" and *Look* magazine carried the story that "The Test-Tube Baby is Coming."[13] A journalist thought laboratory conception posed implications for the 1970s and 1980s as significant as those the atomic bomb had posed in the 1950s.[14] The author of an article in *The Times* of London warned:

The test tube time-bomb is ticking away ... Ultimately we could have the know-how to breed these groups of human beings—called "clones" after the Greek word for a throng—to produce a cohort of super-astronauts or dustmen, soldiers or senators, each with identical physical and mental characteristics most suited to do the job they have to do.[15]

Those wary about bringing together eggs and sperm externally argued that IVF threatened the sanctity of marriage and family, posed psychological and physical harm to the unborn children, would lead to the immoral destruction of human embryos, would make women experimental pawns in research in which men tried to assert control over reproduction, and introduced the senseless creation of people in an era of world overpopulation. It also amounted to experimentation on those who could not give consent (the unborn children), contained no clear stopping point, used scarce medical resources, was not natural, and did not cure infertility.[16]

Those enthusiastic about IVF argued it would spare couples from the psychological trauma of infertility and save them from repeated unsuccessful attempts to conceive in less effective ways, lead to knowledge that would help insure healthy children, and preserve the family by bringing children to those who want them the most. They responded to criticisms against IVF by saying IVF was no more unnatural than caesarean births, should not be diminished merely because it did not cure infertility, posed no apparent risks to children, and was not immoral in that embryos were potential but not actual human beings.[17]

Observers packaged their arguments in literary styles revealing fundamentally different ways of approaching the issue. Critics posed questions in their titles, looked to the future, and assumed a choice:

Babies by Means of In Vitro Fertilization: Unethical Experiments on the Unborn?

Moving Toward the Clonal Man—Is This What We Want?

Shall we "Reproduce"?[18]

Practitioners tended to use the technical language of gonadotrophins, Bavister's medium, zona pellucida, pronuclei, and metaphase chromosomes, and they entitled their articles in the past tense as statements of factual accomplishment:

Human Blastocysts Grown in Culture

Factors Influencing the Success of In Vitro Fertilization for Alleviating Human Infertility[19]

Writers outside the scientific world used images of "neo-Hitlers," "cloned hominids," "wombs for rent," "huboons" (a cross between baboons and humans), and "test-tube babies." Although scientists also expressed concern about the ethical implications of IVF, it was primarily outside observers who looked to the global implications of the technique. Paul Ramsey, a religion professor and a man once described as "formidably disputatious, occasionally pontifical, a master polemicist given to hyperbole, a feisty, occasionally prickly, but always civil critic of the views of others," was one of the more vocal of the critics.[20]

Ramsey, who saw every problem with IVF, and Edwards, who saw virtually no problem, attended the same conference in 1971 where, according to Edwards, Ramsey delivered a critique of IVF with "Gale 8 force."[21] To Ramsey, IVF was "unethical medical experimentation on possible future human beings," inherently immoral, and not in the best interest of the women into whose uteruses the embryos were placed. In vitro fertilization was merely the first step down a road of distasteful applications that would "in foreseeable succession add up to immense disvalue for the human community." Aldous Huxley's *Brave New World* beckoned, Ramsey thought, with extracorporeal gestation (outside the uterus) and genetic manipulations as the steps of the future.[22] The two men represented nearly totally different symbols of IVF, the one seeing it as a promise, the other as a social and moral bane.

Those who wrote of the "thorny" and "prickly" issues of IVF drew attention to its problematic features. Those who wrote of "maximizing implantation rates of human zygotes" drew attention to medical problem-solving. Those who predicted "cohorts of super-astronauts and dustmen" oriented attention to the consequences of IVF; the reporters of scientific accomplishments oriented attention to the importance of valid scientific design. If, in the socratic way of thinking, truth came from the clash of opposites, the stage was well set for an uncovering of the hitherto unknown reality of IVF.

The imagery of IVF took a new turn when the setting shifted from embryos in the laboratory to adult couples who wanted to conceive through IVF. Unfortunately the first attempt was mishandled to such an extent that it did little more than feed the nation's tabloids. The actors were Landrum Shettles, the physician who had published the book showing pictures of human eggs, Raymond Vande Wiele, the head of Shettles' department, and Doris and John Del Zio, a New England couple who wanted a baby.

Mrs. Del Zio had given birth to a daughter in 1963 but internal scarring and other complications left her fallopian tubes irreversibly blocked. She married a second time and her efforts to conceive with her new husband took her from doctor to doctor in search of an answer. Three surgical attempts to clear her tubes, done without anesthesia because of allergies, each ended in disappointment. Three doctors advised her to have a hysterectomy but she persisted with the hope of a pregnancy. "We desperately wanted a child of our own."[23]

In 1973 Dr. Shettles took steps to achieve what he hoped would be the world's first external fertilization of a baby. He arranged for a colleague at another hospital to withdraw follicular fluid that might contain eggs from Mrs. Del Zio. Mr. Del Zio, present at the hospital, was given a test tube containing the fluid to carry to Dr. Shettles, who in turn mixed Mr. Del Zio's sperm with the contents in the expectation that the egg would fertilize.

Apparently unsure about sterilizing the mixture, Shettles asked a neurologist how to do so.[24] She looked at the mixture (later described as a "horrible-looking mess")[25] and informed Dr. Vande Wiele of what Dr. Shettles was trying to do. The department head called Shettles into his office and, in a cloud of fury, confronted him.[26] Had Shettles received permission for this experiment? Had he cleared it with the hospital's human experimentation committee? What experiments had he done to justify this?

Shaken over the implications for the hospital, fearing the hospital could lose its funding from the National Institutes of Health,[27] worried that transferring the unsterile mixture would endanger Mrs. Del Zio's health, annoyed at Shettles for not following procedures, and perhaps carrying a grudge from statements Shettles had previously made,[28] Vande Wiele removed the vial from the incubator and opened the stopper, thus contaminating whatever was in the tube.

This first effort to achieve an in vitro fertilization ended in an emotional turmoil, with Mrs. Del Zio, a woman once "involved with the Girl Scouts, involved with life,"[29] emotionally scarred, and Drs. Shettles and Vande Wiele with a persistent legacy attached to their reputations. It was a measure of public uncertainty about IVF that Vande Wiele was pictured as both hero (for stopping an untested medical experiment) and villain (for destroying what in the public mind was an actual embryo). Mr. and Mrs. Del Zio, whose perceived last chance at pregnancy ended with the twist of a vial lid, brought suit in 1974 against Vande Wiele, the hospital, and the hospital's operators for malicious destruction of their property and for psychological harm to Mrs. Del Zio.[30]

After this abortive attempt, test-tube babydom retreated from the headlines until 1978, when Edwards and Steptoe in Britain announced the first ongoing pregnancy from an external fertilization. Once again, IVF showed its remarkable ability to capture public attention and draw colorful symbolism. Some observers worried about "monster births" and commented ominously, "God knows what kind of baby it will be."[31] Others showed a fascinated anticipation. The expectant mother, Lesley Brown, was monitored by the press to the extent that she literally went under cover in the hospital in the pregnancy's last months.

Meanwhile, the Del Zio case reached Federal District Court in the same summer as Lesley Brown's last trimester of pregnancy. There was cruel irony in the timing of the trial. During the weeks Mrs. Del Zio, once a "happy, pleasant woman," and now a "depressed, crying, overcome, broken woman,"[32] went each day to the courthouse. Lesley Brown in Britain buoyantly awaited the birth of what was destined to be the world's first authenticated "test-tube baby." Newspapers carried the two stories side by side during the summer of 1978, shifting from photographs of a worried-looking Mrs. Del Zio to predictions about Mrs. Brown's anticipated birth. When, in the middle of the Del Zio trail, Mrs. Brown gave birth to Louise Brown,[33] newspapers juggled the headlines of the technique with its many faces. "Shettles They Called It a 'Monstrosity' " blazed on one side of the paper and "For Louise, Mother's Milk" on the other.[34]

Not surprisingly, Louise Brown's birth was, against the worried backdrop of the 1970s, very nearly anticlimactic. A headline in the *New York Times* conveyed a wary relief. "Infant in Britain reported 'Normal.' "[35] The British were not as reticient, trumpeting their newest citizen with pride "And Here she is. . . . THE LOVELY LOUISE."[36] *People* magazine named her one of the ten most important people of the decade by virtue of her mere presence.[37] At intervals over the next years, women's magazines kept track of Baby Louise's growth and gave readers a watch over the child similar to that spanning decades in the life of the Dionne quintuplets.

Two events that summer—the "Test Tube Death Trial"[38] and the Louise Brown "miracle"—brought IVF solidly into the open. With the latter came an immediate step toward the changing of the guard as IVF's critics lost their steam. In this country, an unusually large part of the population—93 percent, according to one poll—had heard of Louise Brown's birth and 62 percent of these people could at least partly explain the procedure.[39] Sixty percent of Americans polled approved of IVF for infertile married couples, and 53 percent said they would try IVF themselves if they were married and unable to have a child by another means. Louise Brown's birth vindicated IVF. One ethicist commented that with the birth, IVF ceased to be an ethical issue.[40]

In 1978 it appeared that Landrum Shettles had not been incorrect in his goal; he had merely been using "Model-T Ford" techniques while Edwards and Steptoe were at work with a 1978 Porsche.[41] When IVF worked, the public turned to the medical community which, in turn, took the definitional lead from the army of pundits that had heretofore been warning of IVF's dire consequences. A subtle shift occurred in which Paul Ramsey now looked merely cantankerous; Leon Kass, who had argued against IVF's artificiality, seemed old-fashioned; and the journalistic headliners appeared to be sensationalists. When Lesley Brown said to Patrick Steptoe, "Thank you for my baby, doctor, thank you," she echoed a broader closure on the uncertainty of IVF's exploratory years. On IVF's coattails came the newly respectable medical subfield of infertility which, as described below, fanned the embers of an evolving set of ideas, symbols, and beliefs. These beliefs in turn justified and created the need for the use of IVF.

THE BIRTH OF A MEDICAL FIELD

With Louise Brown and subsequent births in Australia and the United States came a heady measure of respectability for the long-fledgling subfield of infertility. Infertility had been one of the less popular, if not *"the* least popular," branches of gynecology.[42] For one thing, it lagged behind the combatant ideal of twentieth-century medicine. Whereas doctors in the nineteenth century eased pain and suffering and ministered to the sick, doctors in the twentieth century cured disease. Medicine in this century is "war" and doctors are the warriors who "combat" "invading" viruses and tumors, "fight" death, and "launch" full-scale "attacks" on the sources of illness:[43]

It's an *overwhelming* infection: she's got an *infiltrating* carcinoma; the body's *defences;* he's having a heart *attack; killer* T cells; we must treat him *aggressively* and use everything in therapeutic *armamentarium;* we've wiped out small-pox.[44]

Against the medicine-as-war metaphor, infertility fared poorly. Infertility is not life-threatening; neither, for the most part, is it cured. Rather, infertility treatment turns around diagnosis and circumvention. If the husband has nonexistent or submotile sperm, the treatment of choice in most of this century (apart from adoption) has been to inseminate the wife with a donor's sperm. A baby is born, the purpose achieved, and the husband still has absent or subactive sperm. If the wife does not ovulate properly, fertility drugs stimulate ovulation and a pregnancy hopefully occurs. After the baby is born, the drugs are stopped and the woman reverts to an anovulatory state. As one gynecologist put it, "Infertility is not a respected type of field—be it the male end of it with andrology or the female end of it in gynecology. We think in terms of traditional diseases. If you haven't got a lump, then you are not ill."

Infertility as a field has historically lacked aggression. Its specialists produce babies, if they are lucky, but not a cure. The enemy is circumvented in a truce but not defeated. The very language indicates an absent quality: *in*fertility, *a*novulation, *a*zospermia, sterility. Even the once oft-used term for the infertile woman—barren—connotes bleak images of a parched, thirsty terrain devoid of life. Also, at least 10 percent of the time, no reason for the infertility can be identified. With so-called idiopathic infertility, the enemy is invisible and physicians and patients fight a peculiar battle with guerrilla warriors.

Other difficulties subverted infertility's rise as a field. One was the view that unlike traditional diseases, in which patients sought medical help for pain, sickness, discomfort, or life-threatening disease, with infertility there was a choice. Infertility treatment was seen as a luxury ("to fulfill a wish")[45] for couples who wanted but did not, medically speaking, *need* a child. Theories were also advanced that a certain level of infertility benefitted society by preventing overpopulation.[46] About IVF it was once said, "the development of test-tube babies can be compared to the perfecting of wing transplants so that pigs might fly: an impressive academic exercise which could lead to useful knowledge, but which in itself can only be called unnecessary."[47] Leon Kass wrote that infertility is "hardly a matter of vital national interest—at least not unless and until the majority of American women are similarly infertile."[48]

In the light of population crises in the world, it was not uncommon to think of infertile couples pursuing not just a luxury, but a frivolous one at that. Thousands of parentless children live in institutions. Infertile couples could meet a social duty as well as filling their own needs by adopting a child. Indeed, up to the 1970s, adoption was the method of choice for infertile couples. Told, "don't worry, you can always adopt,"[49] they coped with infertility in nonmedical ways.

Infertility also labored under biases against women that have appeared in various forms throughout history, including the idea that infertility was a "divine retribution for sin," and that women were to blame for infertility because of "excessive luxury, physical work, and intellectual activity."[50] Beliefs that childlessness was invariably the woman's "fault" have pervaded cultures over time. *The Experienced Midwife*, a book written in the seventeenth century, was egalitarian—and unusual—in its tests for infertility, which gave equal billing to woman and man: "To know whether the fault [of infertility] is in the man or the woman, sprinkle the man's urine upon a lettuce leaf and the woman's upon another, and that which dies away first is unfruitful."[51]

More often the woman was presumed to be the cause, or at the least, she was the one subject to "salves, plasters, pultices, inhalations, gargles, pills, suppositories, pessaries, fumigations, douches, and enemas" of every description.[52] In more recent times, instances still could be found of physicians routinely subjecting women to the modern day equivalents of poultices and pessaries—hysterosalopingograms, biopsies, and other equally unpleasant diagnostic procedures—without so much as having tested the sperm count of the spouse. One obstetrician, for example, studied 103 couples who were infertile because of a problem traced to the male partner. Fully 70 percent of the wives had undergone surgery to diagnose the infertility before the husbands were even examined.[53]

Thus, gynecology and its subfield fell under a sway that imputed wrong-doing or fault to the female or at least held her responsible for remedying the infertility. "Every gynecologist is familiar with wives," writes one physician, "who consult him or her about an infertility problem and state that their husbands won't furnish a semen sample for analysis."[54] With infertility's identification as a "women's matter" came the same kind of downgrading as has been historically associated with women's baliwicks.

So too were there assumptions that infertility, as a woman's issue, was a psychological matter. Friends and relatives of infertile couples who advised the wife to "relax" reflected the broader view that infertility was, in many cases, traced to a woman's psychological aberrations. Specialists built varied theories about the causes of psychosomatic infertility.[55] Some studies, for example, averred that psychosomatic infertility was associated with a woman's hatred of her mother and her fears that her child would hate her also or that she would die in childbirth as punishment for her feelings.[56] Although some infertility is psychologically based, it is easily outweighed by infertility with clear physical indications. As one psychiatrist noted:

Two decades ago psychogenic factors were thought to be causative in about 30 to 40 percent of all infertile couples. ... With the development of improved diagnostic techniques and a better understanding of reproductive physiology, a diagnosis can now be established for over 90 percent of infertile couples; through treatment, about half of these can be helped to achieve a pregnancy.[57]

Conditions were little better for the study of male infertility, androl-ogy. The hesitation to look to the male as a partner in infertility was partly based on unease about securing semen samples through mastur-bation. This kind of societal pall caused the discoverer of the "male animalcules" in 1677 to assure the Royal Society in London that he identified them from a sample "obtained during normal conjugal coha-bitation" rather than through a man's unnatural act.[58] In addition, men had difficulty accepting a diagnosis of infertility and resisted seeking help. One advance lay in the ability to freeze human sperm, which led to sperm banking for artificial insemination by donor to circumvent male infertility. Artificial insemination by donor, now known as donor insemi-nation or DI, ran into moral chastisement, however, in an expressed belief, surfacing in a crusty judicial opinion in 1954, that AID was adultery, the wife was the adulteress, and the child the bastard of an illicit union.[59]

21

Several events in the 1960s and 1970s inserted new vitality into infertility as a field. The so-called "humster test" was developed to study male infertility by allowing researchers to cross a hamster egg with human sperm to assess the sperm's ability to penetrate an egg.[60] The laparoscope, an instrument with a light and magnification lens on the end which could be inserted without heating up into a woman's abdominal area to examine her fallopian tubes and detect reasons for blockages, opened diagnostic and treatment procedures for female infertility.[61] Knowledge about hormones, derived from work with birth control pills, advanced the use of fertility pills to hyperstimulate a woman's ovaries.

Barbara Eck Menning highlighted the need for infertility treatment in a book written in 1977 describing the experience of infertility.[62] This brought the topic into the open as a process with stages of denial, isolation, anger, grief, and resolution.[63] Earlier, in 1973, Menning had formed a network of groups known as Resolve in which couples met and talked about the psychological pain of infertility. The open discussion of infertility as a painful process encouraged a recognition of the emotional effects of infertility and the possibility that psychological problems were an effect, not cause.[64] The evolving statement of need for advances in infertility got a push with the Supreme Court's abortion decision of 1973[65] that was widely thought to lead to a reduced availability of babies for adoption. It was after this decision, noted one gynecologist, that infertility became a "red-hot" area.

Against these combined events of books, laparoscopes, and an abortion decision, the efforts of Edwards and Steptoe to circumvent the most common cause of infertility in the woman, tubal blockage, gave scientists tangible material to work with. In vitro fertilization was vivid and dramatic. To mix egg and sperm in a glass dish and to see a cleaving embryo was like making babies. This was a technique of action; it promised results; it expanded infertility from a woman's field to a technique using couples and seemed to offer an answer to male infertility. In vitro fertilization gave to infertility aggressive symbols of medicine. Physicians and technicians in IVF hyperstimulated follicles, aspirated eggs, spun and capitated sperm, cultured and fertilized eggs, and transferred embryos.

In addition, new beliefs and symbols began to take shape with physicians, patients, and sympathetic observers as the initiators. These beliefs define a need and suggest new conceptions as a resolution for that need. Infertility is coming full cycle, from being seen as an unimportant condition two decades ago to having status today as a very important social condition. The stated need revolves around an "epidemic" of tubal infertility and a dearth of treatments for it, a shortage of adoptable babies, and a desperate clientele. The number of visits to physicians' offices for infertility treatment nearly tripled from 1968 (600,000 visits) to 1984 (1.6 million visits).[66]

About the epidemic in tubal infertility, those sympathetic to IVF point out that tubal blockages are the most common form of female infertility and that they account for 25 percent of it. Tubal infertility is estimated to affect between 260,000 and 500,000 American women.[67] It results from scarring from abdominal surgery, ectopic pregnancies (themselves caused by tubal blockages), appendicitis, endometriosis, scarring from abortions, venereal diseases, and pelvic inflammatory disease (PID). One physician has written that PID itself is an epidemic in our society, "secondary only to the common cold":

Of women who have had one episode of salpingitis, 11% to 12% are left infertile; after two episodes, the figure is 23%; and after three or more, it is 54.3%. By 1990, almost 300,000 U.S. women will, it is estimated, have been rendered sterile by PID [pelvic inflammatory disease].[68]

In vitro fertilization is also said to fill the needs of the estimated 1 percent of the 500,000 American women who have tubal ligations for birth control each year and want them reversed, most often because of remarriage and a wish to have a family with a new husband but also because a baby had died shortly after birth.[69] The need for IVF is also couched in beliefs that infertility is on the rise as a result of delayed childbearing and the aftereffects of prolonged use of birth control measures.

In vitro fertilization is thought to be the most logical way of circumventing tubal infertility. It was estimated in 1983 that if one takes into account desire to conceive, age, and other factors, there are 440,000 potential candidates for IVF now existing in the United States, or approximately 36,000 a year.[70] An alternative to IVF, surgery to repair blocked tubes, is successful only part of the time. The success rates for surgical repair of blocked tubes was in 1979 40–50 percent for salpingolysis, 25–40 percent for resection, and 10–25 percent for fimbriplasty.[71] Techniques involving tubal transfer and artificial tubes are, at present, still in experimental stages.[72] In vitro fertilization benefits persons with the following diagnoses and history: "tubal disease unresponsive to therapy, endometriosis unresponsive to therapy, cervical mucus abnormalities unresponsive to therapy, oligospermia, combinations of the above, unexplained long-term infertility."[73]

Another alternative to IVF, adoption, is thought no longer to be an easy alternative. The Supreme Court decision on abortion in 1973, birth control methods, and fewer social restraints against illegitimacy and single motherhood mean there have been fewer Caucasian babies to adopt; indeed, adoption placement dropped from 69,000 in 1970 to 25,000 in 1977.[74]

The need for IVF is magnified by the suggestion that those women who want to conceive but cannot are "desperate" to do so. The women need the technique right away because their "biological clocks are ticking." In the face of the monthly ticks of the body's time bomb, with menopause the explosion, women are "desperate" and are "willing to try anything." In vitro fertilization is a "last chance" and a "last hurrah" for biological parenthood:

My infertility patients are desperate. My in vitro patients are even more desperate. This is their last shot. I have to accept this. Here, with knowledge comes power—the ability to conquer, to give hope where there was not hope.

If you put 100 women over 40 in a room and tell them only one percent will get pregnant, they will beg to be part of that one percent.

These people are willing to try anything.[75]

When the first IVF center was set up in this country in 1981, over 3,000 people signed up immediately,[76] and were apparently unaffected by the fact that no births had been reported here and that the success rate at first (from two births after 100 transfers) was 2 percent.[77] The ones trying first, when the success rates were low, were said to be the elite of the infertile—the ones willing to use the last weapon. One woman described herself as "gutsy" for trying IVF. A nurse coordinator said women who try IVF do not "just stew" about their infertility: "It takes courage to do this."

Thus, new symbols and beliefs arose based on a stated need and a course of action in the medical community. With this interpretation has come a further changing of the guard and with it the power to shape ideas and assumptions about new conceptions. Alfred North Whitehead has written that symbols undergo a "continuous process of pruning and adaptation."[78] The history of IVF suggests that the leadership for that pruning has shifted to the medical sector where, as the next chapter shows, the justification for consumption takes quieter and more detailed shape.

CHAPTER THREE

The Responsible Physician

I n the doctors' offices beliefs about modern use of IVF are defined and order is put on the emerging new conceptions. In these offices the controversial becomes commonplace in the form of rituals, symbols, routines, and language that comes with the everyday practice of basic and expanded IVF. Whether consciously or not, physicians have taken the lead as gatekeepers in the minutiae of IVF. As gatekeepers, they have both fed and limited the consumption of new techniques.

THE IVF CENTER

T he trappings of a business are unmistakable in the medical world of IVF. In 1987 American couples spent an estimated $1 billion on infertility treatment. Seventy million dollars of this went into attempts at IVF, which translates to 7,000 couples paying an average of $10,000 each for IVF.[1] In 1987 169 clinics offered IVF and the related technique of gamete intrafallopian tube transfer (GIFT) across forty states and the District of Columbia. Although some clinics stop offering IVF for want of patients, around ten new clinics begin offering it each year. The number of centers rose from 125 in 1984 to 144 in 1986 and 169 in 1988. Administrators at a start-up infertility clinic reportedly have to invest at least $1 million to become self-sustaining in two years.[2]

The estimated potential clientele for IVF is one million persons and the estimated income will be $2 billion by 1990.[3] Private clinics need a large roster of patients to keep business healthy and they have turned to public relations for help. University centers, which once enjoyed a corner on the market, are facing competition from private clinics that can, unlike university clinics, advertise for patients. University clinics, on the other hand, have the advantage of being able to operate even if patient rosters drop. They are research institutions, and their endocrinologists and embryologists teach their craft to medical students with or without a competitive IVF program. To function efficiently with few patients, centers sometimes close for several months and initiate IVF cycles only at certain times of the year.

University clinics rely for patients on referrals from physicians (often alumnus physicians from their medical schools) and the reputation of their team members built through publications, poster sessions at conventions, and workshops. Private centers use increasingly aggressive marketing techniques in order to create for themselves a "brand-name" as "center[s] of excellence."[4] At least two chains of IVF centers have been set up. Private clinics recruit patients by mass mailings to gynecologists, advertisements in professional journals, and packaged brochures.

One clinic features a brochure in a grey, wine, blue, and brown packet with maps, descriptions of the center's services, price sheets, and a byline on the front page, "Here When You Need Us." Another sends a booklet with colored photographs describing IVF. Its final page shows an 8" x 11" photograph of a woman nursing an infant. Increasingly, centers appeal directly to potential patients, as the center that advertised in *The New York Times Magazine* with the byline, "Now . . . A New Option for Infertile Couples."

The IVF community exudes messages of business and service. A not untypical center has an aura of beneficence to it. Humane touches dot the waiting rooms—walls and carpets of mauve and peach, platters of cookies, coffee pots, and bulletin boards labeled, "Our Babies," with photographs of the center's baby successes splayed in stretch terry suits and propped up on sofas with the parents' "thank you" written on the bottom. Larger clinics hold orientation sessions for patients to ask questions and get to know one another.

The nurse coordinator, a person who is "at heart a patient advocate," stays in daily contact with the patients. Surprisingly often, she (the coordinator is invariably a woman) will have experienced infertility herself and will have insight into the patients' needs. She schedules the laparoscopies, ultrasound tests, and medication distribution and, in general, "wears many hats" as she monitors the flow of patients through the program.

Although the clinicians show the same range of personalities as do physicians of any specialty, a beat of enthusiasm is common. One IVF director who wears a button, "Infertility Is Inconceivable," conveys the hope that is the elixir of childless patients. The physician who laments that his patient's belly looks like "a road map of Kansas" from repeated and unsuccessful operations to clear blocked tubes sees IVF as the last hope as surely as do the patients. "The biggest reward is seeing it work," this same physician said of his interest in IVF. "What fun, what fun." Said another, "When it does work—when they do get pregnant—it is the ultimate ego trip. You feel very, very proud of yourself." In addition: "I love infertility. It has always been my first love. I enjoy seeing people have children. My wife says I am such a narrow-minded Southerner that I want everybody to be just like me—I have children."

Also, on the IVF team are the scientists and technicians (the "real heroes of IVF") trained in andrology (the study of male reproduction), endocrinology (the study of hormones), and embryology. They are the ones who, in the small, windowless laboratories, spin and prepare the sperm, separate oocytes from the follicular fluid brought from the operating room in test tubes, coax the membranous cumulus from around the oocyte, prepare the medium in which the egg will be cultured, mix the egg and sperm, keep watch as the egg matures, and, in general try to replicate as closely as possible the conditions of natural conception.

The need for professional recognition, prestigious publications, partnership in an elite IVF team, and the personal "rush" of the serendipitous discovery all motivate the scientist: "I have always been interested in female infertility. There is such a knowledge explosion now that you are outdated if you are not involved at the core. The perfectionist in me had to know what was taking place. . . . I would say that my colleagues in the in vitro field are obsessive/compulsive. What they need and have is a careful adherence to detail. They must have the perseverance to keep searching for the detail—for that one little thing."

The division of labor varies from center to center. In IVF's early years, embryologists took over many duties themselves: "You find yourself inseminating at 4:00 in the morning, 11:00 at night, and again at 3:00 in the morning. Those seem to be the favorite times for inseminations! I did it all alone for the first eight months. Now three scientists work under me. We rotate the odd hours, although I still make the decision of when to inseminate."

This embryologist was also the clinic's director and the one who broke the news to patients about successes and failures in the laboratory. Saying she was a "laboratory type," and "not a people-relating type," she was

27

relieved when the clinic was well enough established to hire more team members. Although the "egg man" or "egg woman" is less likely today to be known to patients, each is a key to the successful operation of a program:

"I had to talk the physicians into waiting 72 hours [to transfer the embryo]. I was nervous after. I had never taken an embryo to 16 cells. I did not sleep much that night. I know I must have dozed off but it did not feel like it. When it worked out, I felt I should wear a sign saying, 'It worked!' "

"There are many mileposts—when you obtain your first egg, when it first fertilizes, and when it cleaves. Then when you find you can do it over and over . . . It is a personal accomplishment when nature works."

In vitro fertilization has been a technique of incremental advancements nearly as microscopic as the tissues with which the scientists work. The scientists learn what it is like to watch an egg cleave into two parts, then to look again and see it in four parts, and to know that their craftsmanship helped make that happen. They learn the optimum time for fertilization, how long to let the sperm and eggs rest before mixing, and how not to use plastic petri dishes with knobs on the bottom that accidentally catch tissues. Watching, they form hunches and let serendipity play a part. Workshops are held to convey programs and techniques rapidly so that some centers model themselves completely, down to the design and brand name of the last catheter, on established programs. The near-glee of the early scientists gives evidence of the spirit that can be found in an IVF clinic:

"I felt elated when we had our first success. To think that this person is alive because of technology! Cold chills went through my body when I saw my first embryo under the microscope."

"The scientific challenge is gratifying. It is just a tremendous accomplishment. The reproductive aspect is almost glamorous. Creating life in a test tube is almost science fiction."

"It is a new and exciting area in reproduction. It is a clinical application that *works*. It is an extension of everything we do. It is the logical culmination of research and knowledge. I do not see anything new in sight to revolutionize infertility. This is the big breakthrough."

The pulse of optimism, change, problem solving, and pragmatism is similar to that of other high technology fields. There is a certain innocence to it and there are signs of a virtuous intention.[5] At the same time, however, this thirst to improve, refine, and discover has an unnerving dimension to it. There is the danger that visions will take on a momentum of their own and become an end in themselves, with the patient left in the background. A saying among practitioners is that the "baby is the by-product," i.e., that the knowledge gained will be more important than the babies produced.

Here is Robert Edwards exuding that the "whole field is in my grasp" if only he could get eggs.[6] Here are doctors predicting that with IVF "we would bring hope to thousands upon thousands of infertile women and there might well be all kinds of other benefits to human kind" and that IVF "has provided opportunities which if developed with understanding and skill will provide great benefits for society in general."[7]

When the vision becomes an end in itself, that which takes place in the pursuit of the vision becomes secondary. A headline in the Del Zio case charged, " 'Test-Tube Mom Was Pawn in Doctor's Quest for Glory' ";[8] and subsequent efforts to achieve an IVF birth show just how far Shettles had been from an actual pregnancy. Physicians easily speak of the desperation of their patients, perhaps not fully comprehending that with desperation as a motivation, anything is possible in the pursuit of a vision or end. The desperate patient has given the go-ahead to try everything—a heady permission to experiment, perfect, and refine. Interestingly, no studies exist of the possible desperation of doctors and scientists to achieve their goals. Without data, one cannot assess to what extent the desperate patient is actually a projection of the driven practitioner.

The physician treads a fine line with enthusiasm and vision. On the one hand optimism gives the patient hope and the incentive to go an extra step when discouraged. On the other hand it risks raising the patient's hopes inordinately and falsely and it also feeds uncircumspect consumption in which couples pursue goals because they are there to be sought.

How physicians innovate and why, and the impact of innovation on patients and society can be seen by the way they have ushered embryo freezing into normal IVF protocol since 1984. Practitioners have the power to introduce, channel, and control the pace of IVF variations. In the case of embryo freezing, as discussed below, they have moved quietly, quickly, and not always with introspection to produce rituals that are accepted by patients, policymakers, and the general public.

EXPANSION TO FREEZING

An endocrinologist had a ready answer when asked in 1984 what was next on the IVF agenda: "Freezing." Following years of research in which embryos of cows and other species were successfully frozen, thawed, and transferred to the uteruses of the animals for pregnancy, the first successful birth occurred in Australia in 1984. In theory embryo freezing (cryopreservation) offers hope for higher success rates in IVF. When embryos beyond the three or four usually transferred at a time are frozen and stored, they can be thawed for transfer to the woman when she is in a natural state, several months after the stress, anesthesia, and hormonal hyperstimulation of the initial IVF cycle.[9]

With freezing, physicians can control the number of embryos transferred at a time and can reduce the odds of multiple pregnancies (still higher than average with IVF) and risks to mothers and fetuses. As figures become available about the optimum number of embryos to transfer at a time, freezing will let physicians modify their practices to transfer the best number (perhaps eventually one or two) and freeze the rest.[10]

The theory of freezing has enticed a growing number of clinics to offer it as part of their IVF programs. The number rose rapidly to around one-third of the centers in 1987.[11] In 1986 fifteen programs with cryopreservation facilities responding to a survey reported having frozen 824 embryos for 319 patients, with a median number of 2.8 embryos per patient. This was an increase from the 1985 data, in which nine programs reported freezing a total of 289 embryos for 105 patients.[12]

Physicians see freezing as a service to patients. The director of a small IVF clinic without freezing apologized for not offering it: "We are a small program. We need to be larger to do embryo cryopreservation. It is part of the overall service we will like to give to patients. Without it we are offering suboptimal options to patients. We should be offering it. We have decided to offer a more complete range of decisions."

When physicians at one established center went before the hospital's ethics committee to present the case for freezing, the committee members went away persuaded freezing was a needed service for patients. One member of that committee commented, "It is more propitious for the woman. . . . We saw that it was wrong *not* to do it." A member of the ethics committee at one hospital noted that the committee functioned with an "assumption of legitimacy" of freezing:

> "The ideology was to avoid repeated surgeries. They [the doctors] said that there was no risk from freezing embryos—they could screen thawed embryos [for defects]. They said there was less risk to the woman from repeated retrieval procedures. . . . People on the committee raised questions about risks and benefits of freezing but not about freezing itself."

Physicians and staff members see freezing as an emotional boon to patients as well. It will save patients from having to take hormones that make them edgy, travel to strange cities, and undergo laparoscopies. The couples can relax with the knowledge that they have embryos. Nurse coordinators have noted:

> "Patients are *excited* about frozen eggs. They don't have to be monitored or stimulated each time. The way we present it affects their perception. Freezing reduces the odds of multiple birth and it is not costly. It dissipates anxiety if freezing is done. Patients know they have something in the tank. They are happy about that."

> "They will get extra mileage for their money with freezing."

Enthusiastically, practitioners move ahead with freezing, buying the equipment, enrolling in workshops, and contracting with centers to share access to freezing equipment. Directors have many motives for starting a freezing program. Freezing can enhance the program's credibility, attract patients, make the program financially self-sustaining (cryopreservation is not a labor-intensive technique that uses many resources), and bring in storage fees to support other features of the IVF program. The risks appear to be low, it is state-of-the-art technology, and it can buy time for less successful centers by giving them more numbers with which to work (e.g., a director could say, even though the center has had no births, it has a dozen patients with embryos in storage). For the scientists, an added motive is publishable data on methods of freezing and thawing. Predominantly, however, the motive for clinicians and scientists appears to be the faith that freezing will help produce babies.

Because practitioners see freezing as a benefit, they convey this message to their patients. "The way we phrase [the freezing protocol] makes

31

a difference," said one nurse coordinator, and a director noted, "We present it [IVF] to patients and then say we are going to freeze in excess of four embryos." He felt that stating freezing as a given reduced the couple's stress by saving them from having to make an additional decision.

Information sheets and consent forms affirm freezing's assumed worth. In research institutions where freezing is an experimental procedure (this is not always the case—in some institutions it is treated as clinical practice, and doctors do not have to go through review boards to get it approved), patients are told in consent forms they are "invited" to participate in or "selected as candidates" for a research project, and they are assured that their status in the IVF program will not be jeopardized if they decide not to participate. In these forms, the hope of a higher pregnancy rate is couched in cautious but positive language: "[Among the] potential benefits from this study *may be* an increased *chance* of pregnancy occurrence," or "[this is a] technique *we hope* will improve the success rate of in vitro fertilization" (emphasis added).

The potential risks are also stated tentatively:

"We [the wife and husband] understand that these studies of these human pre-zygotes and extensive investigations of cryopreserved animal pre-embryos have not demonstrated a significant increase in risk of abnormalities in offspring that had been cryopreserved."

"Embryo freezing has been successfully used in cattle and laboratory rodents with no known adverse results, but there is very limited experience with human embryos. The risks associated with human embryo freezing, thawing, and transfer are unknown at present."

"Cryopreservation of human embryos has been done without known adverse effects at several medical centers in this and other countries. However, we cannot be certain that there are no risks to freezing human embryos."

As with IVF in general, success rates, at least at the beginning when there were no data available on freezing's successes, were given in general terms with global references:

"The success rate with frozen embryos transferred in the human has not been determined, however the procedure has been utilized in several centers in the world and to date several clinical pregnancies and live births of normal infants have resulted."

"We [the patients] also understand that several laboratories worldwide have demonstrated the ability to cryopreserve human pre-zygotes and to establish pregnancy after transfer. Several normal babies have been born subsequent to the transfer of such frozen-thawed pre-zygotes."

In this quietly persuasive way, freezing became integrated into accepted IVF protocol. In one program, for example, about 95 percent of the patients froze spare embryos. After the program achieved its first pregnancy with a thawed embryo, 100 percent of the patients elected to freeze spare embryos. The lure of freezing is contagious, flowing from doctor to patient. A social worker at one hospital routinely asked IVF patients, "Will you consider embryo cryopreservation?" Some replied that they "just heard about it today." Others appear to go along with freezing without deliberate attention to its implications:

"They [the patients] are thinking about this cycle only. They think, 'Let's transfer the best number and worry about frozen ones later.' They think, 'our hope lies in this cycle.' "

Patients, like physicians, tend to think of numbers as the key to future success. To have ten frozen embryos is like money in the bank. The embryos transferred in the initial IVF cycle are the equivalent of spending money; the frozen embryos are in savings, gathering interest and becoming more valuable.

Yet missing amid this optimism and hope is information from which the patient can make a reasoned choice. The consent forms, with their vague references to risks and benefits, do not give a clear understanding of just how experimental freezing is. Given, there have been several births around the world, the more important questions are: Several births out of how many? How many couples have frozen embryos? How many embryos have been frozen? How many embryos have survived the freezing and thawing? How many embryos that have survived the thaw have been transferred? What is the percentage of births? Is it higher than with fresh embryos?

Also missing from this optimism and hope is a sensitivity to the possibility that embryo freezing may not always be in the best interest of the patient or at least that its effects are problematic and open to debate. In dealing with freezing, what they see as "the best thing in the world," doctors are using with more than a mere medical technique; they are introducing something entirely new to the field of human reproduction. Here, for the first time ever, the genetic stuff of potential human beings is inserted in 1/16-inch straws with a couple's name written on the plug and housed in a barrel-like tank under the counter of a laboratory room. There the embryos stay, out of sight and untouched, for months or years during which time couples think about them and make decisions about them.

Never before has it been possible to store and suspend, over time, human embryos. With time, perceptions change, events arise, and emotions unfold. With IVF in general, it was not known that some women would develop attachments to their embryos by naming them; asking to receive the laboratory dishes in which they were created; marking the anniversary of the embryo's loss; and looking, acting, and thinking they were pregnant after embryos had been transferred. It was not anticipated that with IVF some women would measure their self-worth by the number of eggs they produced or embryos they and their husbands fertilized. External fertilization opens each part of conception to examination, quantification, and measurement. With this novel visibility come new emotions, expectations, and behaviors.

Embryo freezing directs women to even newer uncharted psychological waters. It puts the visibility of reproduction into suspended animation. If a woman bonds with her embryos the day of fertilization, what happens to the bonding when the embryos are stored over time? Does she distance herself from the embryos to prepare for the possibility of disappointment? Or does her mind do subtle things over time and build the embryos so they take on the traits of babies or fetuses? What goes through a woman's mind when she says proudly she has two frozen embryos in another state or when she asks her doctor how her "triplets" are doing? What goes through the mind of a husband who jokes about "freezer burn" or feels vaguely uncomfortable about the safety of the embryos in cold storage? If it is grievous when embryos do not implant during basic IVF, is it more or less grievous when they do not implant after having been stored for months or years?

It is also unclear what goes on in the minds of couples who find they must stop freezing the embryos. The couple may divorce or separate; experience the death of a spouse; face a hysterectomy, premature menopause, chronic illness, or loss of money; run into a limit on freezing imposed by the center; or have a multiple birth, succeed in adoption, or decide to stop trying to conceive. For these and other reasons the couple may be in a position to order the destruction or donation of their embryos. How do they make the decision? Does it bring with it remorse or guilt? How will the couple handle the decision if the wife and husband disagree about what should be done with the embryos?

For something with as many emotional components as infertility, the psychological dimension of freezing is curiously overlooked by physicians eager to start offering cryopreservation. When practitioners are asked about possible emotional dilemmas of freezing, they readily suggest that the nurse coordinator or hospital psychologist would be in a better position to talk about that. It is a topic of little interest or concern, as evidenced by the fact that a computer search of all medical and nursing publications four years after freezing started revealed no studies dealing with the emotional implications of freezing or of decision making by patients trying freezing. Further, a physician writing a detailed summary of the IVF process in a medical journal included a short paragraph on the emotional aspects of IVF that differed noticeably from the tenor of the rest of the article with several caveats that "in my opinion" the emotional elements ought to be examined.[13] Whether the author included the caveats because of the dearth of empirical studies or because of pressure from editors, the implication was the same: the emotional elements of IVF are treated warily by medical professionals.

Anecdotal evidence suggests that freezing may, indeed, pose varied dilemmas for patients. Freezing can interfere with closure of the infertility experience. Patients often know when they have "had enough," and may not welcome finding out that a center will let them go through IVF more than three or four times. Similarly, when they reach the stage of satiation, the presence of frozen embryos can interfere with the decision to withdraw. A woman at one center, for example, decided she had had enough when, as a last straw, she lost a chance at embryo transfer because the hormonal stimulation did not work. This meant waiting several more months, undergoing stimulation again (for some women, drugs are needed to prepare their uteruses for the transfer of the thawed embryos), and gearing up for one or more future failures. Her wish to get out of the infertility roller coaster was stopped, however, by the presence of four frozen embryos. She thus stayed on the infertility track even though emotionally she had reached her limit.

Freezing can also lock patients into treatment at a single hospital. Some clinics refuse to transfer embryos to other centers. One woman with polycystic ovaries who ended up with ten frozen embryos began, however correctly or incorrectly, to lose confidence in the program. She felt she had to stay with the physicians, however, because that was where her embryos were. When encouraged to talk with staff members about her feelings of anxiety, she refused because she feared jeopardizing the status of the embryos if she expressed anger toward the hospital.

In short, when left to themselves to administer embryo freezing (and

35

basic IVF before it), physicians define the matter as a medical issue and deal with patients correspondingly. When they consider freezing's advantages and disadvantages, they look to medical matters, downplay the emotional components, and show a seeming lack of curiosity about emotional facets. This happened with basic IVF, now it is happening with freezing, and, one can expect, will occur in future variations of expanded IVF. New conceptions are rounded techniques with social and psychological implications pushed, too often, into the square pegs of a medical world.

MAKING DECISIONS

Freezing is a case study in how decisions are made within the medical community about matters doctors define primarily as medical matters but that have strong emotional, psychological, and societal underpinnings. Doctors and scientists are trained in making decisions about the technological dimensions of treatments. The embryologist, for example, collects data about embryo freezing, contacts colleagues about methods, talks about freezing at professional meetings, and publishes results of experimental protocols. It is thus ironic, given the prizing of empirical data for decisions about how to freeze embryos, that much less attention is given to policies about administering the embryo freezing protocol.

Assume, for example, the IVF director decides to add freezing to the program. A freezer, storage unit, liquid nitrogen tanks, and other supplies will be ordered; a technician specializing in animal or human embryo freezing will be hired; permission will be received from the hospital administration; and team members will make arrangements to visit another program, which will serve as consultant and model. What then?

The Freezing Protocol. Embryos can be stored indefinitely, it is thought, perhaps up to hundreds of years. What will be said to the patient? Will the center freeze the embryos for as long as the patients want? Or will they put a limit on it? Unlimited freezing certainly keeps options open and it saves physicians from destroying embryos. On the other hand, it raises the prospects of cross-generational transfers, interferes with a patient's closure, and may put physicians into an unwanted offshoot of IVF of the "long-term storage business." If physicians put a limit on freezing time, what should that limit be? Should it be two years? Perhaps a couple will not be able to use the embryos within two years. Should it be an option to extend the time for consecutive two year periods? It would make business sense to ask a couple to pay storage fees at regular intervals but time extensions put the center back into the storage business. Should it be five years? Most patients would use embryos within that time. But what if the patients need an extra year? Should that be granted? Or should the limit be the reproductive life of the woman?

How should a physician decide about the length of time? Is it important to place the hospital's interests first (limited time might be safer from the legal standpoint inasmuch as no one really knows whether embryos can safely be stored for years and years)? Or is it important to place the couple's interests first? Might not the interests of the potential child be important lest children are born after embryo donation with genetic parents long since dead? Or how about societal interests? The longer the storage the more likely embryos will be forgotten by couples or not used and be available for trafficking, which would conflict with interests expressed against commercialism in the public debate.

When setting up a freezing program, should the physician charge patients? Charging would help finance the program and research connected with it. On the other hand, with freezing experimental, is it ethical to charge patients for that research? Should clinics wait until their success rate has improved to charge? If they decide to charge, what is a reasonable fee? A one-time charge? A per year charge? The same fee for all embryos? Should they just cover costs (e.g., $350) or charge more in order to reinvest it into the program (e.g., $1,000)? Should the storage fee go up along with the cost of living? If couples later donate the embryos to the center, should the patients be reimbursed so they will not end up paying the center for its research material? Or would this look like selling and buying human embryos?

Should the center offer donation of embryos to other couples if the original couple decides not to use the frozen embryo themselves? This would prevent the destruction of embryos. On the other hand, some directors report that couples are willing to donate embryos but not to receive them, which raises the prospect of unused and unwanted embryos. In addition, it may raise dilemmas for couples who do not conceive and who have donated embryos. Might they wonder if the other embryos did implant and are now their genetic children living with other parents?

A review of centers offering freezing shows an array of practices and policies. Some university clinics either do not charge for freezing or they plan to charge after having their first birth. Those that charge ask from $350 to $500 and even up to $1,000 or more. All give their patients choices about what to do with unwanted embryos. These choices involve combinations of (1) destroying the embryos, (2) donating the embryos to research, or (3) donating the embryos to other patients. Alternatively, couples may elect to have only a certain number of eggs fertilized, which means there would not be extra embryos and freezing would not be used. Some allow patients to name the recipient, others do not.

On the matter of timing, centers variously freeze for two years, five years, ten years, the reproductive life of the woman, or impose no limit. Most centers use consent forms asking patients to spell out what should be done in the event of death or divorce. Other administrators eschew detailed consent forms, saying they are probably not legally binding in any event and the physicians would rather take matters as they arise.

On how to reach the decisions, one director admitted that "we were working in the dark." The criteria are primarily nonmedical and they are infused with notions of trial and error and simple arbitrariness. On the length of time, for example, directors have said:

"We freeze for five years. We have limited facilities. This is an arbitrary number. We reached it after advice from the legal department. It seemed like a reasonable amount of time."

"We will freeze for five years. Some on the [hospital ethics committee] wanted two years; others the woman's reproductive life. So we compromised on five years. I looked at the case of one couple who had twelve embryos. Five years will give them a chance of two pregnancies."

When asked to rank factors influencing how they made decisions about IVF policy, directors of clinics put their own discretion and judgments of the IVF team in the highest positions.[14] They also use models presented by colleagues with whom they have worked or whom they respect at other centers. About embryo freezing policies, for example, IVF team members have said the following:

"We got input from the University of Washington. I was at UCLA so we used that. We also used Houston; one member of our staff is from there. The nitty-gritty was based on these three programs."

"We modeled our program after Fairfax, Virginia. It was modeled after Australia. We used the Virginia program because it was the most academic and had a large program geared to this research. The consent form was modeled after the program in Cleveland. It was a more exhaustive form. Lawyers, philosophers, and others were involved with it. I was impressed with the careful scrutiny."

"We modeled it after USC—[Dr.] Marrs. Completely. We patterned the entire program while [the Director] was at USC with Marrs."

"Tacoma, UCLA, Virginia—we got copies of the consent forms of everyone else and we'll take the best of them all."

After a time, individual centers have emerged as the pioneers after which other centers modeled their policies so that new centers and others trying to improve their programs attended workshops to learn the techniques. Not only do they copy the model's recommendations down to such details as the brand of freezing unit and the number of cells the embryo should be at the time of freezing, but they adopt socially relevant policies about how long to freeze and what to put in the consent forms.

Administrators at hospitals with ethics committees might consult the committees when setting up embryo freezing programs, but the role of the committees seems to be more to react than initiate. Said a member on one ethics committee: "had I wanted to nitpick, I would have been out of place." Members of the ethics committee at another hospital variously said of the freezing decision: "our function was to document the process" of having consulted the community before making decisions about embryo freezing; the director was not "wringing her hands" waiting for the committee to give approval; and the committee acted as a "sounding board" for the physicians. Committee members suggest ways of clarifying the language of consent forms; their role as policymakers is less substantive.

Another form of internal review, the Institutional Review Board (IRB), is helpful only in hospitals that have an IRB and where the IRB members regard freezing as an experimental protocol needing approval. The director of one IVF program noted that: "[The IRB members] were concerned only with clinical research on patients. They didn't even want to review [the EC program] because they thought it wasn't research. They thought it was clinical application only."

The American Fertility Society guidelines on freezing are used rather sporadically. Although the short 1984 ethical guidelines of the AFS (approving cryopreservation as ethically acceptable, among other things) have been called the "bible" of IVF directors, the lengthier 1986 guidelines,[15] complain directors, came out too late, after programs had been set up. Others who claim to have read and used them are unable to cite where the guidelines helped. One director expressed the opinion that "directors are not going to roar to their libraries to get copies of the AFS guidelines" in order to set up their programs.

The upshot is that ad hoc policies about freezing and other IVF variations such as tissue donation and egg freezing are often made without specified or consistent criteria. Instead, they are made on the basis of the director's discretion, informal talks among colleagues, and modeling across programs. Ethics committees tend to be used secondarily to justify and clarify, which leaves medical personnel as the referents of policy. Decision making takes place within IVF centers and reflects the perspectives of scientists and clinicians.

These decisions count, however, both for the patients and for society. The steady growth of freezing gives tremendous leverage to the medical community. The daily activities of freezing (and of basic IVF and future variations) amount to ad hoc policies that are idiosyncratic when taken individually but significant when taken together. Physicians build options, rituals, language, and images and, in so doing, they make freezing mundane. These ad hoc policies then set the building blocks for public awareness and beliefs about working with stored embryos. Practitioners are among the first to put order on a dramatically new technology. They are gatekeepers who inadvertently control the passage of ideas about techniques to the broader public. The minutiae of IVF have an impact greater than the sum of their parts. To the practitioners intent on getting babies for infertile patients, the nonmedical implications of freezing are not especially interesting, important, or obvious.

What is the embryo? One emerging routine with a societal impact is a working definition of the embryo. There is much discussion in the literature on the status of the embryo. To members of ethics commissions here and abroad, it is a potential human being worthy of special respect. To physicians, it is a collection of cells with specific properties depending on the embryo's developmental stage. To couples, it is a powerful symbol of hope and potential parenthood. It is a tangible sign the husband's sperm and wife's egg can unite and it might be the closest thing to biological parenthood the couple has experienced.

Of all the things that the embryo can be—of all its biological, symbolic, and social "personalities"—the one that emerges in the daily administration of IVF and cryopreservation is the legalistic notion of the embryo as property. This was anticipated in the 1984 ethical guidelines published by the American Fertility Society, in which the embryo was said to be the property of the couple: "It is understood that the gametes and concepti and the property of the donors."[16] The need to clarify this in writing in individual centers became clear with the case of the Australian orphaned embryos, in which the couple whose embryos were stored were killed in an airplane crash.[17] The resulting lawsuit and controversy warned practitioners that storing embryos opened the door to legal quandaries if no one had clear responsibility for the tissues.

Thus, the technique of freezing created the need precisely to define the embryo. Labeling the embryo as a legal entity may be little more savory to medically minded physicians than recognizing a couple's emotional attachments to embryos, yet freezing's complexity demands a legal dimension. One hospital lawyer stated: "The physicians were concerned with patients' care. They thought it was the best thing in the world to have frozen embryos. I, as a lawyer, was concerned with institutional liability. What if something should happen when embryos were moved? What if the couple should divorce? I was concerned with the implications of the actions. They were concerned with benefits to the couple."

The language of the embryo-as-property bears little resemblance to the embryo-as-human language of persons opposed to alternative conception (see chapter 6). "Embryos that are frozen and stored for you are your property," couples might be told in consent forms, "you are the owners." Couples signing up for IVF and deciding to freeze any spare embryos sign a preconception agreement that can be likened to the prenuptial agreements arranged by engaged couples in a divorce-minded society. Couples are asked, even before eggs are fertilized, to provide for the disposition of potential embryos in the event of death or divorce.

The agreements have been known to overwhelm and turn away couples wary about IVF in the first place. The consent forms contain the following kinds of "legalese":

"In the event of divorce, we [the wife and husband] understand legal ownership of any stored pre-zygotes must be determined in a property settlement and will be released as directed by order of a court of competent jurisdiction."

"Based on currently accepted principles regarding legal ownership of human sperm and ova, we have been advised that each embryo resulting from the fertilization of the wife's ovum by the husband's sperm shall be the joint property of both of you, as the wife and husband, who are deemed to be the legal owners."

The language of property, disposition, and discarding brings with it a new kind of depersonalization—not the grandiose depersonalization of the early years of "test-tube babies" and "cloned hominids" but of a less theatrical and more understated type. It is easy to forget, with talk of "test-tube babies," that one was working with living infants; it is equally easy to forget, when talking of "disposition of property" that one is working with the stuff of a potential human being. Moreover, it encourages embryo bonding when couples are asked, before the embryo is even created, to take responsibility for it:

It is our intention that any embryos not used in an effort to initiate a pregnancy in _____, the wife, for any reason be disposed of as follows:

1. That the embryos be donated for use by other infertile couples, if otherwise permitted by applicable law, Hospital policies, and the ethical standards referenced in this Form:

YES____   NO____

2. That the embryos be utilized in research projects permitted under Hospital policies, the ethical standards referenced in this Form, and applicable legal requirements:

YES____   NO____

3. That the embryos be disposed of in accordance with Hospital policies, in a manner consistent with the ethical standards referenced in this Form, and applicable legal requirements:

YES____   NO____

Arguably, this bonding weds couples to the process of IVF by enhancing their sense of reward. It might also worsen the sense of loss if embryos do not implant. Thus, communication between doctor and patient is hindered if the one sees neutrality when talking about the embryo and the other holds intense feelings about the embryos.

What Is the Relation Between the Couple and Embryo? A second routine emerging in the medical community is the daily definition of the relationship between the couple and the embryo. Couples are not "parents" in the traditional sense inasmuch as embryos are not "children." They are "owners" as stated in consent forms, but the ownership is different from ownership of furniture or automobiles. What, precisely, is the relationship between couple and embryo? What are the couple's rights? What are their limitations? The relationship falls between the cracks of existing law and invites a revision of civil codes to take the new techniques of IVF, freezing, and gamete donation into account. In the meantime, the working principles are initiated and nurtured in the IVF community.

In theory, as expressed in the 1984 American Fertility Society ethical guidelines, couples have the "sole discretion" to make decisions about their embryos. This model imputes authority to the couple and, in so doing, mirrors existing codes and legal decisions that grant couples wide, though not unlimited, control in making medical decisions about their offspring. In practice, though, the couple's autonomy over their embryos is not so far-reaching. Consent forms in freezing programs, for example, warn that "relevant legal and ethical standards" or laws, judicial decisions, and hospital policies take precedence over a couple's autonomy. The law on what can and cannot be done with embryos is unformed and inconsistent,[18] and these caveats give little guidance about what couples can do in regard to their embryos.

The "sole discretion" principle is also limited by specific restrictions written into consent forms about a couple's authority to make decisions about embryos. Centers variously limit couples from taking embryos to other centers, naming the recipient for donated embryos, transferring embryos across generations, or transferring large numbers of embryos at once if that is against hospital policy. Clinic administrators reserve for themselves the right to select recipients for donor embryos, decide what will be done with embryos donated for study, dispose of embryos from couples who do not make payments, not transfer embryos thought to be abnormal, put time limits on embryo freezing, and close down freezing facilities.

Physicians are legal pioneers trying out basic principles about what is and is not permissible in the odd kind of "parenthood" a couple enjoys with its embryo. It is not known how much autonomy couples should have vis-à-vis their microscopic gametes or what tests and criteria should be used to weigh the interests of the couple, physician, embryo, and potential child. Using abortion law as a guide, one would suggest that the couple's authority over the embryo, which is less developed than the fetus, would be great indeed. Yet governmental restrictions are not really at issue here. Instead, controls are placed by the hospitals. In some cases it appears that hospitals are more cautious about what should be done with embryos than are patients. Thus, in the absence of legal standards, physicians define the wife's and husband's authority to define "treatment" for their embryos.

Discarding the Embryo. A third area in which physicians hold the power to shape ideas and rituals is the matter of the embryo's loss. If the language of what the embryo "is" ventures into new territory, the matter of what the embryo is "not" goes even further into that terrain. If the embryo is not "alive" in the sense of being fully human, neither does it "die" in the sense that a human dies. Where, then, does one turn to describe the embryo's end? Does it "expire"? "disintegrate"? "not survive the thaw"? Administrators show uncertainty about the language of the embryo's demise. Some are blunt; their consent forms contain clauses about the option of "destroying" or "discarding" embryos. Others skirt the issue; their consent forms refer to embryos being "disposed of" or "thawed and not allowed to undergo further development." The consent form at one center states that "embryos will be disposed of" and then adds in parentheses, as if to clarify, "(destroyed)." Another explains that "you should be aware that embryos thawed and not transferred will not develop further."

The physician walks a fine line between accuracy and sensitivity. On the one hand, it is sensitive to speak carefully about the loss of embryos that have come to mean something to patients. On the other hand, clouded language may obscure the reality of the choices for patients. It may also set the stage for secrecy on activities in IVF centers. Already studies are being conducted abroad where wording about the creation and destruction of embryos for research is so obscure it is difficult to tell what has taken place.[19]

The matter of embryo destruction (as opposed to embryo loss that follows inadvertently from failure during IVF) has been the subject of many socially based concerns. Irrespective of the validity of those concerns (some would say embryos are simply collections of cells—no more, no less—and destruction of them poses no ethical problems), it is important to understand that basic notions about embryo destruction are being shaped in IVF centers. The language reveals uncertainty among practitioners themselves about embryo destruction. It also shows that something that has raised concerns is now starting to sound regularized and routine. It is not uncommon to see in consent forms, for example, that "embryos will be disposed of in a manner consistent with professional ethical standards and applicable legal requirements." There are no legal and ethical standards about disposing of embryos, however. When asked how an embryo might be disposed of ethically, practitioners are often momentarily speechless, ready with a joke, and then able to come up with an answer: letting the embryo thaw and disintegrate naturally rather than throwing it in the wastebasket or washing it down the sink. The language and method of disposal is thus in the hands of individual practitioners who are not immediately cognizant of their power as gate-keepers of societal morality.[20]

The justification for disposal is also in the hands of the physicians and scientists who rank and evaluate embryos. Embryos that are not transferred because they do not look good (they are morphologically unsound) are said to be "defective," "abnormal," or "nonviable." Those that are morphologically sound but not needed by the couple are "unwanted," "spare," or "excess." In research studies abroad, embryos used for study are "unsuitable for embryo transfer," "spare," or "reject" embryos.[21] They are graded on scales by their morphological soundness.[22]

ASSUMING RESPONSIBILITY

When freezing first came to public attention, observers warned it would raise many ethical dilemmas. Among other things, they warned it would raise "disturbing," "extremely difficult," "thorny," "enormous," "incredibly complex," and even "nightmarish" issues and questions. Today, fewer than five years later, freezing is being quietly integrated into IVF protocol. On the one hand, this understatement may be an accurate depiction of freezing's impact on society. On the other hand, today's relative silence about freezing diminishes public concerns to near somnambulism. The language, symbols, and routines being shaped in the medical centers where freezing and IVF are increasingly taking on the aura of normalcy are not correct or incorrect. They are simply an emerging belief system or way of putting reality on something new under the sun.[23] Perhaps even more important than the substance of the emerging beliefs is the method by which it is being done—subtly and without much oversight.

What is happening with freezing is thus an example of what will happen with future applications of IVF. Increasingly, it is being left to the private sector to shape routines. In the technique of ovum transfer, in which embryos are flushed from one woman's uterus and transferred to the uterus of the intended gestational mother,[24] the quiet is exacerbated by efforts of its pioneers to patent the procedure. In the matter of embryo research, now going on "quietly" in Britain[25] and other countries, silence is also a feature of decisions about how embryos will be studied and why.

With embryo research, symbols and language are also emerging. The metaphor is directional; research on embryos (and corresponding clinical applications) will take us "up" a path of increasingly positive applications including improvements in IVF, prevention of genetic defects, treatment of genetic defects while at the embryonic stage, and the understanding and control of adult diseases.[26] Next on the horizon are embryo biopsies, for example, in which parts of embryos will be cut off for chromosomal analysis and the "parent" part will be frozen until the test results are known. If analysis (karyotyping) shows no obvious defects, the frozen embryo will be thawed and transferred to the patient.[27] This "antenatal" diagnosis preempts even the "prenatal" diagnostic tests of amniocentesis and chorionic villi sampling.[28]

Already we see a pulse building for new applications that go beyond infertility treatment. Apart from the scientist's excitement in pursuing new knowledge and the physician's enthusiasm in applying it, one must remember that each technique creates yet another group of experimental subjects and emotional pioneers. What kinds of choices will couples have when their embryos are biopsied? Who will help them come to grips with their choices? Will the human side of choice be lost amid the glamor and promise of the technique for future generations?

The image of the physician brings with it notions of virtue, caring, and the doing of good for the patient. Beneficence has origins in the Hippocratic Oath which requires the physician to declare under oath that "I will apply dietetic measures for the sick according to my ability and judgment; I will keep them from harm and injustice."[29] The patient is tinged with vulnerability in the doctor/patient relationship, and the doctor's role is imbued with the expectation of trust.

In the IVF setting the patient's responsibility is to make informed choices; the doctor's responsibility is to provide information so the patient can make these choices. The word "doctor" comes from the Latin *docere,* to teach.[30] The sharing of information is inherent in the doctor's role as one who helps the patient understand. This includes giving statistics about IVF at the doctor's center as well as at other centers. It also means communicating uncertainty when appropriate. Freezing, for example, is an experimental procedure with unknown effects. Too little is known about the emotional correlates of freezing to gauge accurately what the beneficent act for the patient really is. The physician trying to anticipate the patient's best interest might keep in mind that the interest is still unknown. Beneficent doctoring in this case would be the sensitive communication of uncertainty.

Responsibility means treating each patient as an individual with unique needs and a unique history of infertility. There is wisdom in the counsel that "patients are, first of all, persons, and only secondarily patients to the physician's ministrations."[31] Treating patients as persons means individualized care. It also means avoiding the desperate patient stereotype and substituting in its place a presumption of rationality. Where desperation is apparent, it ought to be recognized for the extreme condition that it is; its presence should signal extra reserve, not permissiveness, by the physician. Desperation should turn on an orange, not green, light, and indicate the need to bring social workers or other hospital personnel into the decision process.

Treating patients as persons means helping the patient see alternatives to birth as the IVF resolution. If the patient's overall health is to be achieved, the physician can help coordinate the search for a "positive good" for the patient if conception does not occur.[32] The physician can also arrange follow-up contacts with patients who do conceive and who return to their usual obstetrician for care during pregnancy. There are indications that when infertile women do get pregnant, some may have trouble coping with success after years of struggling with failure. They may delay bonding with the fetus and be confused and feel guilty about discomfort during pregnancy or post-partum depression.[33] Physicians who take women into uncharted psychological waters thus act responsibly if they make sure their clinic offers help during and after IVF.

The responsible physician will take seriously the making of ad hoc decisions within her or his center and will be sensitive to the impact of seemingly mundane decisions on patients and society. Deciding whether to freeze for two years or five years or the reproductive life of the woman is not an arbitrary decision. It makes a statement. For the patient, it puts a closure on attempts to conceive. For society, it says something about the relationship between couple and embryo (two years is not much of an ownership, for example). Thus, physicians are virtuous gatekeepers when they keep in mind the impact of decisions they make. Likewise, the language of discarding embryos also makes a statement. Couched or euphemistic language inures society to something about which concerns have been voiced. Arguably, it sets the stage for dissembling when future embryo research is conducted. If the need to dissemble exists, the practitioners have moved too fast for society to keep pace. Embryo research is appropriate when the language of destruction can be articulated clearly and without shame.

In making those decisions, the responsible physician will have specified criteria in mind. Leon Kass has written that the doctor as physician (and "not merely a body technician") "must also be a knower of souls, those of his patients and, not least, of his own."[34] There are different models of applying medicine,[35] all of which have validity and all of which are used by physicians, depending on their own philosophies. The important thing in the ethical analysis, however, is that physicians have an idea of which ethical models are at work. The best safeguard against exploiting the vulnerable patient, writes one ethicist, "is always a combination of a virtuous physician dedicated to the patient's welfare and an explicit and orderly system of ethical analysis."[36] In this way of thinking, the method of researching a decision is at least as important as the substance of the decision itself.

The responsible physician will see IVF as more than a medical matter. It is tempting to evaluate IVF on numerical data such as the rate of egg retrieval, fertilization, cleavage, implantation, and the number of frozen embryos. Yet costs and benefits to the individual's emotional well-being ought also to be weighed. Among other things, IVF and its variations can raise unexpected dilemmas of choice. One learns, for example, from the couple who had decided to donate their frozen embryos to another couple but then had a baby through IVF and changed their minds about what to do with the frozen, now unneeded, embryos after they saw what the embryo could become. Their experience made them see donation in a different light, as something akin to giving up a child for adoption. So too did they see discarding in a new light, as a kind of abortion. Beneficent IVF means being aware of these quandaries so support personnel can help counsel patients in the future. The beneficent IVF protocol will integrate nonmedical components into its sweep as it continues its move into expanded offerings and choices.

The responsible physician will have the courage to draw lines in the administration of IVF. How enticing it is to be able to think, "Surely the whole field was then in my grasp—cows, sheep, monkeys—and man, too"[37] or to understand that "with knowledge comes power—the ability to conquer." It goes against the beat of our culture and economic ideology to draw lines against the consumption of new techniques. It does not, however, go against the beat of virtue to say "no" in order to save couples from unnecessary disappointment, dashed hopes, spent money, and perhaps lost years that could better be spent in alternative ways of coping with infertility.

One French researcher, who views freezing as a way for practitioners to get research material, decided to draw the line in his personal behavior: "Freezing of human embryos is my last venture. I will not go further; I will not try any other 'first.' "[38] Physicians who limit their own consumption are aware of their place in the context of a medical era in which the "triumph of technique" flames a "proliferation of desires, which in turn breed the further growth of technology needed for their satisfaction."[39] It takes courage to say "no" when one is in the heart of the dynamic medical field of alternative conception today. The physicians, too, can become victims of the pressure to consume. By expanding too far too fast they lose centers, patients, and control over what might have been their first love of helping couples with simple IVF:

> "It is difficult to be a physician today. There is pressure to be scientists as well as clinicians. The scientists are not so interested in patient results as in moving ahead from the scientific standpoint. If a clinician gives a paper on induction of ovulation at a professional conference and lists clinical problems based on 1,000 patients without research, people think the person is second rate in the field. If a scientist gives a paper based on scientific inquiry based on five cases, then this is OK."

It takes courage to refuse to admit patients with questionable infertility or to limit the number of times a person will be allowed to try IVF. It takes courage to tell women who do not respond well to ovarian stimulation or women over the age of forty that their odds of conception through IVF are so low as to make their attempts near folly. It takes courage to resist starting a freezing program until the success rates and safety record demand that freezing is really in the patient's best interest. In an article entitled "Baby Craving" in *Life* magazine, couples told of calling centers around the world to find a physician who would transfer their embryos to surrogate mothers and of being turned down by cautious practitioners.[40] It takes courage to say no to a variation of IVF that is seen as an answer; the physician who told the couple it was a "wild" idea came across as the odd person in the article. After all, the couple was dedicated and wanted a baby. Does not the physician have an obligation to help the wife and husband have a baby?

Yet the prevailing ideology defines courage as saying "yes" and pioneering ahead rather than saying "no." Did Landrum Shettles show courage in mixing sperm and egg without systematic preliminary research? Or was it arrogance? Did Robert Edwards show courage in devising a "sperm chamber" in IVF's early years in which he inserted living sperm (presumably his own) in the uteruses of fertile women to capacitate the sperm before withdrawing them for IVF studies?[41] Or was it arrogance? Is it courage and bravado that marks the scientist who would say about trying to perfect IVF, "We discussed other details of how we would proceed. Ethical concerns hardly entered into our conversation"?[42] The responsible physician can better practice humility when the profession itself values humane (which may well mean slow and traditional) applications in the doctor's office.

Physicians are, in their daily interactions and decisions in IVF clinics, the earliest policy builders. Their language, symbols, methods, and rituals put an undeniable imprint on how techniques are integrated into the societal idea of reality. As gatekeepers for IVF and embryo freezing, physicians have the obligation to comprehend the implications of what seem to them to be mundane decisions. Whether these techniques will be a public good or not depends on the acts and presumptions of physicians in the clinical setting. Where they adhere to notions of virtue in presenting choices to patients, are cognizant of their own values, and make decisions in an ethically defensible way, an important step is taken to integrate the techniques into society in a way that will promote their promise.

In vitro fertilization in itself is neither warm nor cold, humane nor dehumanizing. The practice puts the character on it. The yearning to find the "last detail," to add to the list of "Our Babies," and to search for knowledge "of interest to future generations" must not be done in such a rush that the implications for patients and society are lost in the wind.

CHAPTER FOUR

The Responsible Patient

The word "patient" comes from the Latin *patior-pati*, "to suffer, to bear something." In this traditional sense, the patient is a petitioner, a supplicant, a "human in distress, and an especially vulnerable human."[1] In the world of IVF we can expect a special kind of vulnerability resulting from the hype of high technology, IVF's money-making prospects, and the after effects of a couple's struggle with infertility. We can also expect that as time passes and more is learned about IVF, we will see a growth of the patient's autonomy.

Over ten years have elapsed since Lesley Brown displayed a particular type of vulnerability when she said of her role in being the first woman to give birth following IVF: "I don't remember Mr. Steptoe saying his method of producing babies had ever worked, and I certainly didn't ask. . . . It just did not occur to me that it would almost be a miracle if it worked with me."[2]

This chapter asks two related questions: In what ways are patients vulnerable to exploitation in the IVF setting? In what ways can they enhance their autonomy within that setting? In an era of expanded IVF, the patient no less than the physician, policymaker, and general public, must assume responsibility in building a pattern of circumspect consumption. Although technically the couple is the "patient" in this chapter, unless otherwise noted, the patient is assumed to be the female partner. She undergoes the more intrusive physical aspects of IVF; moreover, IVF is more often the treatment for female than male infertility.

VULNERABILITY IN THE IVF CLINIC

The Jaded Patient. It is commonly thought that women come to IVF clinics vulnerable from a prolonged struggle with infertility. From those who write and tell about it, the experience of infertility is indeed harrowing, frustrating, isolating, and generative of self-loathing and blame. It is a "war" in which the possible causes for the inability to conceive are eliminated, one by one. If a diagnosis is reached, available treatments are then tried, one by one. During all of this the woman turns inward, to her body, and the wife and husband together turn inward, to themselves and away from a broader world of children and parents.

Symbolizing this isolating struggle is the temperature chart, which is the first thing to greet a woman upon awakening in the morning. Here, in an effort to find out if she is ovulating properly and to identify the most fertile time for sexual intercourse, the woman takes her basal body temperature for three minutes each morning before doing anything that might prevent an accurate reading. She does not sit up, drink water, or do anything more strenuous than reaching for the thermometer. One woman has written, "Every morning for months, I lay in bed, taking my temperature, afraid one of my two Afghan hound puppies would leap on the bed, demand attention, and raise my temperature."[3]

After taking her temperature, the woman plots it on graph paper and, like an apprentice, learns to detect the slight drop and rise on the line graph that signals imminent ovulation. Temperature taking can go on for months or years, thereby entrenching the habit of looking inward: "I have plotted temperature charts for months and months and months and months"; "Some patients have been taking daily temperature readings for eons." Infertility is the first thing she thinks about before facing the day. It precedes even the morning stretch.

The temperature charts also notify couples of the best time for sexual intercourse and reduce even that act to a "job" or "duty" to be done at just the right time. Couples learn what scheduled intercourse does to warmth and spontaneity. As one woman told it, her husband hissed in anger that he was "no goddamn stud service!"[4] Even couples with the gift of humor find it taxing to meet during the day for an act of scheduled sexual intercourse, sandwiched between the working schedules of each, so the wife can visit her physician, who will, in a post-coital test, take a swab to find out if a property of the cervical fluid prevents sperm from entering the uterus.

Temperature-taking and post-coital tests are apertifs that, along with sperm analysis, occur early in infertility diagnosis to rule out causes of infertility such as anovulation, allergic reactions, or a problem in the way the couple make love. When physicians eliminate simple causes, they move to more invasive medical procedures. Among these are multisyllabic tests like the hysterosalpingogram with its injection of blue dye through the cervix and into the uterus and fallopian tubes. The tubes show up as solid and white objects on the X-ray and reveal blockages in the tubes.[5] The hysterosalpingogram is mildly uncomfortable if the tubes are open; the discomfort is more pronounced if they are blocked.

In diagnostic laparoscopies, the woman is put under general anesthesia and a tube is inserted into her belly so surgeons can inspect her fallopian tubes and ovaries for blockages and scarring and can try to clear them. Sometimes the husband's sperm is belatedly tested and it is found that a low sperm count had been a contributing factor all along. Other times one thing adds to another to produce a condition of infertility with several causes. One woman, for example, had an irregularly shaped uterus due to her exposure as a fetus to diethystilbestrol (DES), a drug her mother used to stave off a miscarriage. Added to that were problems with ovulation and, later, a high white blood cell count in her husband.

A constant sense of loss threads through the infertility experience. Infertility means a loss of the potential for the dreams of childbearing: perpetuation of the family's gene pool; company when the couple ages; joy of a child's presence; the need to nurture; affirmation of femininity, masculinity, and the couple's validity as a pair; and the satisfaction of having control over one's life. Partners who are oriented to pregnancy feel losses connected with that experience: not feeling the physical changes of pregnancy, not enjoying the attention that comes from being pregnant, not being able to breastfeed. Partners oriented more to children feel different losses more keenly: the loss of the role of parenthood, an absence of "passage to adulthood," or the inability to relive one's own childhood.[6] They even lose the ability to grieve properly:

Death before life . . . before we even knew our child, because he never existed. The hardest part of this kind of death is the fact that it is the death of a dream. There are no solid memories, no pictures, no things to remember . . . . He never existed.[7]

Barbara Eck Menning writes that the grief for infertility is "strange and puzzling:"

The rituals society has for death pertain to *actual* losses, not *potential* losses. There is no funeral, no wake, no burial, no grave to lay flowers on; and family and friends may never know. The couple often grieve alone.[8]

Infertility itself is a loss which brings with it specific losses. Ectopic pregnancies, a not uncommon accompaniment of tubal blockages, occur when egg and sperm unite in the fallopian tube and the embryo cannot make its way to the uterus. Barricaded from the journey it is supposed to make, the cleaving egg attaches itself to the tubal wall and begins to grow. The fallopian tube, two times as thick as a strand of human hair and without the elasticity of the uterus, is an inhospitable substitute for the womb. The cleaving egg grows in the tube until it causes pain or bursts and the woman faces emergency surgery. A tubal pregnancy is a net loss on the balance sheet, destroying a healthy or partially blocked tube, and sometimes an ovary too. A potential child is also lost, thwarted by the inopportune place in which the fertilized egg nestled.

Miscarriages are common for some women, such as those over forty and those having a so-called T-shaped uterus. Women liken the loss of a fetus to a death in the family. The woman bonds to the fetus in early pregnancy. As the only one who has felt its presence, when the miscarriage occurs early in the pregnancy she tends to grieve for its loss alone. Her spouse tends to grieve more when the miscarriage occurs later in the pregnancy, after he has felt the fetus and seen it on an ultrasound screen.[9] A miscarriage brings with it the loss of a formative, potential child. When women are asked how many children they have, they include miscarriages in their calculation.

Couples compare infertility to a roller-coaster ride of fluctuating emotions. The emotional highs build around the heady emotion of hope, the lows around the onset of the menstrual flow and with it a lost chance of pregnancy. Hopes follow lows in a monthly procession.[10] Infertility takes women inward, from the temperature taking to the anxiety over menstruation until their lives are "ruled by the menstrual cycle."[11] Joan Liebmann-Smith notes that the woman is "constantly monitoring her body . . . Every time she goes to the bathroom she checks to see whether she is bleeding or whether her cervical mucus is ripe."[12] With its unresolved answers and constant stress, infertility is the most upsetting life experience (more than the death of a relative) some women have gone through.[13]

The lack of control, frustration, and diminished self-esteem alienate the couple from other people. The struggle to resolve infertility takes on a life of its own. "No amount of discomfort is too much" in the effort to have a child and the willingness to endure discomfort is sometimes exacerbated by guilt over the infertility. Getting pregnant becomes "the most important goal in life, even if [the woman] was ambivalent before."[14] After a time, couples add to or even shift from their search for a pregnancy to the equally frustrating "search for an answer." Couples can spend years "in a wasteland of suspended animation" that can be so draining they have tubal ligations or vasectomies to end the uncertainty and ensure they will not get pregnant.[15]

Some couples, faced with the options for circumventing infertility, find that making choices about these options is in itself a way of asserting control. Women who make the decision to fight the infertility amass experience that takes on the character of a curriculum vita:

"I have had five ectopic pregnancies. The last three were life-threatening."

"After three months of trying to get pregnant I had a miscarriage. That was four years ago. I've been to all kinds of doctors and have had histograms and the works. I've also had three abdominal surgeries."

"We have been trying to conceive for six or seven years. I've had three laparoscopies and one laser laparoscopy to cut the adhesions around my tubes."

As a result of this legacy of infertility, some women come to IVF depressed, with low feelings of self-worth,[16] and dependent on a physician's suggestions about what treatment is desirable. When this happens, women open themselves to a paternalistic interaction with the physician. With paternalism, which has a long-rooted and not necessarily harmful history in medicine, the physician as expert decides, on the basis of her or his judgment what treatment is in the patient's best interest.[17] When the physician acts in the patient's best interest he or she uses the ethical principle of beneficence.[18] The patient as supplicant accepts the recommendations and does not request detailed information about alternative treatments.

It is essential to recognize that the above picture of infertility and its legacy paints an archetypal picture based on the stories of those who tell it and of those sympathetic to new conceptions who want to publicize a psychological pain that has long gone unrecognized. Infertility, after all, was ignored until fairly recently and the infertile themselves were in 1978 called in one account "one of the most neglected minority groups in America."[19] It is understandable that the emotional cost of infertility be publicized as part of an effort to educate the public about a heretofore largely hidden problem. Still, the picture of what might be called the "jaded" patient cannot fairly be generalized to the IVF clientele as a whole.

The Less Jaded Patient. In order to illustrate the diversity of couples who try IVF, it might be useful to distinguish between first wave and second wave patients. The first wave included those who had struggled with infertility silently, before it became a thriving medical field. When IVF hit the headlines, they hit the telephones, trying to get on waiting lists of the first centers to open. Like Doris Del Zio, they had tried everything, which in the 1970s was not much, and their menopause did, indeed, approach like a ticking clock. For them, IVF was the last chance. Even those who had come to grips with their infertility hauled out their mental resources to try one more thing before saying they had done it all.

In short, the popular image of a desperate, aging woman for whom IVF is a last chance has merit, but only to a point. As physicians found out, the early rush to try IVF was followed by a receding number of patients, as the first wave passed through and out of the IVF arena. Couples now thinking of trying IVF are among a second wave who will benefit from better statistics about IVF, more streamlined protocols, and the luxury of relative youth. For these patients, IVF may very well be among the first chances, not the last chance. They do not put all their hopes in one technique, which arguably lessens their dependence on it. These comments by two women illustrate:

> "I've tried everything short of adoption. Now there is the ovum transfer in California. That is asking a lot of another woman. Still, ovum transfer is the closest [to biological parenthood] because [the fetus] would be developing in my own body. I'd give birth to the baby."

> "We will consider surrogate motherhood . . . Sometimes the surrogates want to keep the baby. I'd have to keep in my mind during the whole pregnancy that she may keep the baby. We would have to counsel her all the way through."

This type of patient is less desperate for IVF because she, who lives in a time of growing options for infertility, sees alternatives to IVF. This does not mean she will be free from desperation later or get hooked on another treatment, but it does reduce the prospects of repeated unsatisfactory attempts at IVF that come when women go through a full cycle nine or more times or try unsuccessfully eighteen or more times to get beyond the hormonal induction stage.

In appreciating the diversity of IVF patients (and thereby questioning the popular image of desperation), one can also look to couples who come to IVF centers with secondary infertility. Women with secondary infertility have had at least one child and then became infertile either accidentally or deliberately through a tubal ligation. They differ from women with primary infertility who have never given birth. Doris Del Zio had secondary infertility; she had had a daughter, but scarring after that birth left her infertile.

Arguably, there is less public sympathy for women with secondary infertility, which partly explains why their experiences are not widely publicized. In addition, at least in the early years of IVF, clinicians were not eager to call attention to births to women with secondary infertility because the births seemed less of a miracle and because detractors could argue that the women's tubes may not have been totally blocked. Patients with primary infertility also feel less sympathy for those with secondary infertility:

"Of the first four women in the program, three had had children. I was resentful at first. I did not think this was fair. I wondered, "Why are *you* here?" If some of the others had gotten pregnant and I did not, it would have been a stab."

"It surprised me that in my group I was the only one who had not had children. The others had already had children. They were wives and mothers. This seemed to be their way of filling time. They wanted to have children again. They seemed to be asking, "What else is there for me to do?" One woman had three children and nine foster children. It was curious to me."

Secondary infertility can approximate primary infertility in the feelings of anger and frustration it brings about. According to one woman, "I had a daughter when I was twenty. Since then I have had five tubal pregnancies. I feel like I have been cheated. I just want a second baby."

In other cases, women appear to be nearly blasé about their experiences. One woman, for example, jokes that her friends used to call her the "rabbit" because she had three children in quick succession. After the third birth she divorced, had remarried, and wanted a family with her new husband, who is childless. Her friends think she is "crazy" for paying $4,000 for IVF, but her husband is pressuring her to have a son to carry on his family's name. A woman with four children, now in a remarriage, tells a similar story: "It is not fair to my husband not to have a family. We will consider surrogate motherhood or adoption if this does not work. One way or another we are going to have a family."

Also in the "less-than-jaded" category fall women whose commitment to conception is limited. Cheryl McCartney lists some motivations expressed by patients seeking infertility care:

"I want my tubal ligation reversed so I can give my second husband a baby. I'm sure he would like it, and I know his mother wants grandchildren. For myself, I wouldn't have any more children. I married my first husband, whom I dislike, because I was already pregnant, and then I had a second baby soon after that. I am relieved that those kids are finally in school."

"I am supporting the family because my husband lost his job. If I get pregnant, he would have to look for work and take care of us."[20]

Finally, some women come from the legacy of infertility with strong psychological defenses. One study showed that in a sample of patients who went past the initial visit, most had Ego Strength scores within the normal range.[21] Other women have set ideas about their own limits and how many times they want to try IVF. They are used to disappointment and are aware of their limitations. They are determined to "say 'whoa' " even if the physician does not.

In summary, a range of persons with varied backgrounds come to IVF centers. Some are vulnerable, others are not. Some are desperate, others are not. One can predict that as infertility treatment gets more successful, publicized, and done early in a patient's history of infertility, the desperate patient will decline in numbers. Whether the pervasive myth of the desperate patient will also decline is another matter.

THE IVF EXPERIENCE

For the jaded and not-so-jaded patient, the experience of IVF itself can create a vulnerabilty. If infertility is an emotional roller coaster, IVF is the most intense roller-coaster ride of all. First-time couples come to IVF centers little prepared for the emotional turmoil of the substages of treatment. They expect the large stages—ovulation, laparoscopy, embryo transfer—but they are not always prepared for the way each step within these major stages magnifies their hopes, fears, losses, and rewards. Some come prepared for disappointment at the end—not getting pregnant—but little prepared for the many things that can go wrong early in the procedure. Others come persuaded they will walk away pregnant. Once at the center they come to realize the tension filling the hours between the initial blood draw and the embryo transfer. "It is not like going to a podiatrist,'" said one patient, "it is a major inconvenience. You have to shut down ten days of your life. It is emotionally draining. It is not a minor inconvenience."

At the center patients experience tension about the range of possible snags. At the ovulation stage, the patient rises early in the morning to drive to the hosptial for a blood draw. If she is trying IVF in her home town she fills the day with her normal activities. If she has taken leave from work or is in a strange city for the IVF (often alone, if the husband will travel to the center only for the surgery), she waits. Late in the afternoon she waits to receive or make the telephone call with news about the blood draw results. If the results show she is responding (nearing ovulation) to the medication, she will receive more medication and the next morning will drive once again to the hospital for a blood draw, and wait again until the late afternoon for the telephone call with the results:

"I have been here one week. At 8:00 a.m. I have a blood draw, then I call at 3:30 or 4:00 to find out what to do next. The rest is waiting. The stress level is fantastic. You worry a lot, you're in a strange place. There is nothing else to do but think and worry about it. I am alone. My husband was here for the weekend."

"Waiting is the hardest part. I was there [in the city] for ten days. I was so tied up I did not even want to leave my [hotel] room. I was up and down depending on the blood tests. I played solitaire for five to six hours straight. I never play solitaire!"

In the last three days of monitoring follicles are examined with ultrasound. By this time the stakes start to creep up. Energy and costs have been put into the process. Might the process be stopped? Up to 40 percent of the patients in IVF's early years had their IVF cycles stopped early, before the operation, because their blood draws were not appropriate or the follicles were not the right size or number. Today induction leads to satisfactory follicular growth 65 to 75 percent of the time, which means from 25 to 35 percent of the time it does not work.[22] The solution lies in developing a hormonal combination appropriate for each patient. For some women, the "poor responders," the ovulation induction stage of IVF is never mastered. The tension of the early stages is, feel women, magnified by the hormones themselves:

"My emotions were out of control. I was tired, excited, and nervous. The drugs affected my hormonal level and with it my rationality."

"The drugs changed my body cycle by eight days. I was more hyper, more emotional, less negotiable, and more sensitive. The whole thing was emotionally draining. Hormones make you feel a little odd."

Eventually an injection is given that allows physicians to schedule the egg retrieval surgery for the expected ovulation thirty-six hours later. For the patient this means more waiting and worrying that the eggs will be released prematurely or that the surgeons will not be able to get around the obstructions and scarring of the tubes. After surgery there is the waiting to see if eggs are retrieved (around 90 percent of the time they are) and following that the waiting to hear if the eggs fertilize and then to hear if the eggs cleave normally to the four or eight cell stage.

During this time, the male partner experiences his own tension ranging from concern about how to be helpful to anxiety about producing a semen sample. To reduce the latter anxiety, some centers have special rooms with magazines, encourage the wife to be present if problems arise, or freeze a sperm sample from the husband ahead of time as insurance against an inability to ejaculate:

"After the laparoscopy there was a slight snag. My husband could not produce. He tried two times. The first time just fluid came out. There was no sperm. Finally, they told him he could go home and try. He drove home from the hospital and then went to sleep! The hospital called and woke him up. They were wondering what happened to the sample. He got one at home and then drove back."

After the embryo transfer the couples wait to find out if there is a pregnancy. Even this, with the possibility of a false (chemical) pregnancy, can bring a cruel failure. The more usual disappointment lies in the lack of a pregnancy altogether or the miscarriage of that pregnancy, occurring in approximately 23 percent of the pregnancies.[23] Although the pregnancy rates have risen from the 1 to 2 percent in IVF's early years, they remain low for any single IVF attempt. A 1985 survey showed that doctors performed 7,000 laparoscopies in the IVF centers responding to the survey, which resulted in nearly 900 ongoing pregnancies and nearly 400 births. Translated, the birth rate from the point of laparoscopy was 5.5 percent.[24] The compilers used pregnancies in progress at the time of the survey to predict an ultimate birthrate of approximately 8 percent. If one were to count births from the stage of ovulation induction, the rate would be far less. If one were to count births from the stage of embryo transfer, the rate would be higher.

Counting pregnancy rates is a technical matter which takes into account who answers the questionnaires (the new centers generally have low rates and the established centers have higher rates), from what point in the IVF cycle the birth rate is calculated, how pregnancy is defined (clinical, not chemical, pregnancies are of interest to patients), and whether pregnancy or birth rates are calculated. For the first time, a central Registry is beginning to report outcomes,[25] leading to the conclusion that birth rates are improving but that many patients are disappointed during the IVF cycle.

The IVF experience uniquely opens up each step of the reproductive process to quantification, measurement, and evaluation. Patients feel disappointment if something goes wrong at any step because they have invested energy, hope, and money into the process. Likewise, they experience joy and excitement when each step proceeds smoothly. The emotions are linked to the visibility IVF gives to the reproductive process.

At any one time, American women of reproductive age are either developing follicles, releasing eggs, or having within themselves cleaving embryos. Aside from the phantom feelings of ovulation and the recognizable signs of an imminent menstrual flow, however, they are not aware of the process nor do they feel responsible for it. With IVF, in contrast, each stage is open to counting and evaluation: the blood's estrogen counts, the growth of follicles, the number and quality of eggs, and the number and quality of embryos. This visibility magnifies the feelings of looking inward that started with the infertility experience. When IVF proceeds well, it gives the women whose ego and sense of femininity has been buffeted by infertility an affirmation of self-worth:

"I did so well. I produced so many eggs."

"I feel so good about my body. I really didn't know if I was developing eggs or not before I came here. I was excited to hear about the number of follicles. I was progressing and doing such a good job!"

"I feel pride from having five eggs. I feel more like a woman now."

When IVF is stopped early, however, the occasion for self-blame arises. Women come to IVF centers not trusting their bodies, feeling that the bodies are deficient, abnormal, and silent saboteurs: "Why, I'd wonder, why aren't you doing what you are supposed to be doing? Why? At the end of each month I'd cry, get angry, and ask, 'why?' "

. . . one client spoke about feeling so bad about herself that she stopped going to her athletic club so that other people would not see her body in the locker room. Her body image reflected the defect she felt inside, as if her internal problem of infertility was an external blemish.[26]

Patterns of self-blame reappear and compound as women take responsibility for the outcome of the follicle count, the egg count, and the embryo count.

"Women in the program are so hysterical, so excited. You'll hear them walking down the hall saying 'Oh, I know I'm producing a lot of eggs today' or 'I wonder how my eggs are doing.' It sounds like the Easter Bunny is coming or something."

"I felt touchy about talking about the number of eggs with other women in the program. There was a feeling of competition among them. I had a feeling of inadequacy—am I going to be up to snuff?"

If not handled with enlightened talks with psychologists, nurse coordinators, or other staff members the IVF experience can be emotionally devastating, especially if ended early. When eggs do fertilize and cleave, a symbolic point or affirmation is reached. The embryo is a powerful symbol of hope and, to some couples, the embryo may be the closest thing to biological parenthood they have experienced. A bond grows: "There is only one egg but it is mine." Patients will name their embryos "preemie" or "little one," call to ask about their "twins" or "triplets," and ask for the glass dish in which the eggs and sperm united as a memento. If IVF does not work, they mourn the loss of the embryos. If it does, the couple feel they have known the child before the point of conception: "It is a funny feeling looking at not even a new born infant but . . . the basis of life [the egg], I guess. To know your child even before the egg is fertilized would be a truly intimate thing."[27]

The embryo transfer itself may be filled with the symbol of what the embryo represents, with the couple expressing dreams about its future. After the embryos are transferred, a woman is, mentally at least, pregnant:

"If you have an embryo, you look and act pregnant—you *are* pregnant. The infertile woman is left with so little to work with. The embryo makes it more tangible."

"[W]hen patients have had a transfer, they leave here with a pregnancy in mind. If it does not work, emotionally they call it a miscarriage. They have something to grieve about. This makes it easier. Also, for a short time they were pregnant. They pat their bellies, maybe even name the embryo. They *feel* pregnant."

Often IVF is easier if the woman goes through the point of embryo transfer, where, at least, the outcome is out of her hands. The process has worked, and she has learned about her body and the hormone combination for use if she tries again. Her investment in travel and money and hope will have been worth it:

"If the hormones don't work, it's me. Early failure is more personal. If [the embryo] doesn't implant, I have no control over it. That makes it easier."

"The first time I did not stimulate. This was very hard. I hadn't expected it. I was worried about whether the embryo would stick in my uterus. You can imagine what it was like when I was told I could go home on the fourth day. My ovaries were not developing. It was very devastating."

In summary, whatever feelings of low self-worth, anger, guilt, and frustration that have their roots in the infertility experience can be magnified by the IVF experience. Those women who go through it easily, find answers to their infertility, and, best yet, become pregnant, are the lucky few. More often than not, problems appear and the unprepared woman amasses evidence against herself. The patient need not be vulnerable supplicant, however. Instead, with the guidance of IVF staff members and her own self-awareness, she can become a more discriminating consumer of these techniques.

ENHANCING PATIENT AUTONOMY

The model of autonomy is a more recent ethical model of patient/ doctor interaction which differs from the paternalistic model. As a model, it places authority in the hands of the patient to participate in treatment decisions. Edmund Pellegrino defines autonomy as "respect for the patient's moral right to decide for himself and the physician's obligation to respect and enhance that decision."[28] For autonomy to work well, the patient must have access to information in order to give informed consent for one treatment over others. The authors of such books as *Our Bodies, Ourselves*[29] call for greater autonomy for women in the making of medical decisions about their bodies. In this day when women question unnecessary hysterectomies, radical mastectomies, and caesarean sections, autonomy is a model of note.

In the context of IVF, patients can enhance their autonomy by accepting alternative resolutions from IVF and by taking responsibility for gathering information about the procedure. In each case, practitioners at individual clinics can help or hinder this effort. One factor in the choice of an IVF clinic, then, should be whether the staff members are willing and able to help the patient exercise autonomy.

Alternative Resolutions. Women can avoid the status of desperation if they have alternative resolutions in mind when trying IVF. The desired resolution is, of course, an ongoing pregnancy. If that does not occur, the patient can either continue trying in an unlimited quest with IVF and its variations or can look for other resolutions from the experience and call it quits when pregnancy does not appear likely. The latter is the path of circumspect consumption. It works only if the patient finds a reward short of pregnancy from the experience.

One alternative to pregnancy is to be able to go away from the clinic saying the woman has tried what she set out to try. This means going to the center with an early closure in mind, thinking IVF will be a turning point, a "last hurrah," or a signpost of "getting off the infertility train." A number of women who tried IVF unsuccessfully and then quit have expressed closure as an outcome:

"I felt I owed it to myself, my husband, and to the Lord to try everything. If I didn't try I would never know."

"I was thankful there was one more thing to try."

"You have gone through so much already; it is silly not to go through one more step."

"My concern was that I would have regrets down the road if I didn't pursue it further."

It takes some resilience to stick with closure and it seems to help to have in mind a certain number of attempts before trying IVF. Without pre-set notions of what one is willing to try, the lure of "just one more time" begins to take hold, and the patients become like the conquering Spaniards in South America looking for the legendary El Dorado, or city of gold. Group after group of Inca Indians, the legend goes, told the Spaniards the city lay "yonder," and the Spaniards gathered their seeping energy to trudge over yet another hill to be told once again that the city lay "yonder." Each "yonder" in the reproductive terrain offers a glimmer of hope; at the same time, it reduces the odds the patient will get any reward from IVF. The need to have in mind one's own limits is illustrated by the recommendation among some physicians now that four attempts at IVF is optimal. This has escalated from earlier recommendations of three attempts.

Ideally, the patient will have in mind the optimal number of attempts before trying IVF, but couples may introduce their own limits after trying it one or two times. One woman, for example, tried IVF three times, but with each attempt something went wrong. The first time she did not respond to the medication, the second time she ovulated prematurely and the surgery was canceled, and the third time surgeons retrieved one egg but it did not fertilize. After having said she would try it as often as it would take, she had decided that the fourth time would be her last: "I won't go back. Surgery makes the problem worse. They won't be able to retrieve eggs again. The last time they were lucky to get even one egg. I had so many adhesions. They just had to do it blindly."

Another resolution if pregnancy does not occur is to gain satisfaction from having answered questions about infertility. From the experience couples, for whom everything has gone wrong up to IVF, can see a reason for the troubles or can see that some features of IVF did work well. A woman can learn what combination of hormones works for her, the extent of tubal scarring, and, perhaps, that her eggs and her husband's sperm can unite. She learns about her own commitment to resolving infertility, which may not be as strong as she first supposed. She learns that she can experience a great disappointment and still come out emotionally strong.

A third resolution comes from having faced infertility and talked with other couples about it. Patients have said the following:

"It's worth it to have met the other people. It was helpful to see ordinary people with the same problem. They are normal, friendly. I appreciated that."

"You talk with patients about things you would not even talk about with your parents. We have common feelings. We have already gone through crushing disappointments. We can empathize. Victories are celebrations—feelings of mutual excitement. There is empathy among the husbands too. Everybody understands. It's like having been through a war."

Ideally, couples reach their own alternative resolutions from unsuccessful IVF. As one couple wrote about IVF, "As tough as the odds may be, no one should come without hope: no one should leave without gain."[30] Inasmuch as this does not always happen, sensitive staff members can help provide that guidance. One nurse coordinator, for example, tries to help patients come out of IVF stronger than when they went in. She suggests they use IVF as an opportunity to learn more about themselves, to be aware of their motives for trying it, and to come to an understanding of how much of their lives they want to devote to infertility resolution. "How much energy, money, and emotions do you want to devote to this?" she asks patients. "It is important to be a happy person. Will this help?"

The importance of a supportive context for IVF is increasingly recognized by social workers as a necessary part of an IVF program. A growing body of literature suggests patients should be helped before, during, and at the conclusion of IVF to develop coping skills for IVF's tensions and for reaching alternative resolutions.[31] Ideally, the physician, too, will help patients put closure on their experience. One physician writes that physicians can do this in infertility care by telling patients, for example:

"The in vitro fertilization has cost the two of you a great deal in dollars and emotional distress. Let's make this next trial our last one."

"The amount of healthy tube available for microsurgical reanastomosis is so small that I think I would have only a 5% chance of success. With these odds, I wouldn't advise surgery."[32]

Thus, the dynamic works both ways. In some cases physicians fail to help patients put closure on their experience. In other cases, however, physicians recommend closure but the patients push for repeated treatment. Both doctor and patient bear responsibility for putting limits. The inherent inequality in the doctor/patient interchange, however, suggests that the possibility for exploitation (trying IVF repeatedly when there is no realistic hope) is a constant danger in the IVF setting. The patient can be alert to high salesmanship when signing up for a program. Success rates are only one criterion for selecting a program; humane and low pressure treatment are others.

The patient can ask if the center has counseling facilities. Counseling helps patients through the process; it also helps them put an end to their infertility experience. In vitro fertilization is "emotionally exhausting" and the "end of the road" for those who, if it does not work, "simply have to face their infertility."[33] The patient can also look for self-limiting statements by the program, such as an information sheet stating that only couples with documented infertility will be accepted or that the center will limit the number of times it will start an IVF cycle with any one patient. Another sign that the program is discriminating about its use of IVF is the presence of staff members willing to ask a couple about motives for trying IVF and possibly attempting to dissuade the couple if it appears they are trying to conceive for "inauthentic" reasons. A patient's willingness to undergo repeated and hopeless IVF might reflect unrelenting anger or guilt, as the case of a woman who, through counseling, saw that she was trying through IVF to "replace" a fetus she had aborted fifteen years before and who, with the aid of the nurse coordinator, stopped trying IVF.

Gathering Information. An important key to the ability of patients to participate in the making of rational decisions about IVF is to have access to information about the technique. The less than jaded patient wants information: "I can't hear the chances often enough. I like to hear realism. I don't like to go into things blindly. I want to know what the problems actually are. 'Twenty to thirty percent' does not mean so much. I want to know, 'In X case this goes wrong; in Y that goes wrong.' We patients get to be minor experts at this."

For the patient, securing accurate information can be a hard task.

Right at the start, she is confronted with the IVF myth of the 20 percent success rate. Rarely does one read about IVF without seeing in the same article a reference to the 20 percent success rate. This global figure, called "peculiar" by one physician, is stubbornly repeated and embraced as accurate by the patient and public alike. In vitro fertilization clinics repeat it, as in the brochure published by a center that had had no pregnancies: "The successful pregnancy rate reported for a normal human menstrual reproductive cycle is 10% to 20%. This is very similar to the success rate for IVF procedures, according to experiences reported by medical centers around the world."

The message here, and one likely to be picked up by a patient who is not forewarned, is that 20 percent of the women who walk into this clinic will walk out pregnant. An added, and equally misleading, message is that if she tries four times she has an 80 percent chance of having a baby. Several things make this smooth message misleading. First, the 20 percent figure glosses over vast differences among centers. New centers rarely have pregnancies during the first six months of operation or for the first dozen patients. Other centers have one or two pregnancies out of dozens of clients. By 1987, one-third of all centers had never had a birth; two-thirds of all the IVF births in this country had occurred in fewer than ten centers.[34] The range of success rates varies from zero at many centers to 30 percent at a handful.

Second, as discussed earlier, the 20 percent figure uses the embryo transfer as a denominator; i.e., it is based on 20 percent of the women who make it all the way through the IVF cycle to embryo transfer. Many patients do not get that far into the cycle, however. Up to 40 percent are "canceled" from the cycle before the laparoscopy because they do not respond to the medication. To illustrate, of every one hundred women who sign up for IVF, forty will be sent home early for not responding to the medication. Most but not all of the remaining sixty will go on to embryo transfer. Along the way two or three will have laparoscopies but surgeons will not retrieve usable eggs. Another five will have eggs that do not fertilize or cleave properly. Of the fifty or so of the original one hundred women who reach embryo transfer, 20 percent (10) will get pregnant. One or two will miscarry. Eight of the original one hundred will give birth. The birth rate is 8 percent if one uses the point of sign-up as the denominator.

The realization that many things can go wrong before embryo transfer surprises many couples signing up for IVF. One woman who had flown to the center of her choice only to find out the success rate was around 6 percent said she "freaked out" and would not have tried IVF, given the time, energy, and financial drain, had she known more about the odds. Another said of her first IVF attempt: "When I got to the center and found out that nearly one-half of the patients at that center did not go on to surgery, I became a nervous wreck."

A second misunderstanding (or misrepresentation) comes from different ways centers define a pregnancy.[35] One can distinguish between three kinds of pregnancies: a chemical or "false" pregnancy, in which the chemical tests show a pregnancy but the woman is not pregnant; a clinical pregnancy, based on ultrasound viewing of a twelve-week fetus or observed fetal heartbeat; and an ongoing pregnancy that results in a birth. Some centers count chemical pregnancies in their success rates, which can be misleading to the patient who, after all, is not interested in false pregnancies. Physicians advise patients to ask not about pregnancies but about births. Even then, the possibility of misrepresentation is raised if the center counts twins or triplets as two or three births without saying they were born to the same woman.

A third thing that works against full information for the patient is the unwillingness or inability of physicians to give figures about who gets pregnant and who does not. Women go to IVF centers with dramatically different histories of infertility. Some, like the woman mentioned earlier whose friends called her the rabbit, do not have a legacy of infertility. Supposedly, she ovulates properly, her menstrual periods are regular, and the scarring from her tubal ligation is fairly "clean." Other women have had long and detailed histories during which their tubes have been exposed to repeated surgery, they have taken powerful drugs at various points, and they may have multifaceted infertility. One woman, for example, tried IVF after having imbedded intrauterine devices on two occasions which left her with "massive adhesions" around her tubes.

Another woman had had one child, one miscarriage, and a total of fourteen surgeries, including five during IVF. Still another had a long history of ectopic (tubal) pregnancies, which tremendously damage fallopian tubes: "Both my tubes were damaged at age eleven with an appendectomy. I was pregnant two times—both ectopic. The first time I had internal bleeding for two weeks. I was in the hospital. The tube ruptured. That was the end of that tube. I had reparative surgery and did get pregnant but it was ectopic on the other side. The tube is there but it is not good. I have to get it fixed before I go back [to the IVF center]."

For a woman to make a fully informed choice about whether and how many times she should try IVF, detailed figures about how many people get pregnant with histories similar to hers are essential. One highly educated woman bitter about the lack of information suggested, well before physicians were publishing such information, that: "People should be given accurate information. It is such an inexact science. They need a profile of women who actually do get pregnant. They need to collapse all patients across the country and get data."

Early in the IVF years, physicans tended to publish information about how success rates varied by medical protocol. They asked: what combination of chemicals is optimal? what number of cells should the embryo have before being transferred? how long should we wait between egg preparation and fertilization? They found, for example, that pregnancy odds were best when two to four embryos were transferred at a time.[36] The clinicians paid less attention to the women with such questions as, what women are most likely to conceive?

With more information now available, it is clear that features of the patient do make a difference. The woman's age counts heavily: one study showed more IVF births for women between twenty-five and thirty-four than for younger or older women.[37] Women over forty have been found to have so many spontaneous abortions after conceiving in IVF that some physicians recommend not even trying IVF on women over 40.[38]

Studies have also shown that women who try IVF repeatedly have diminishing odds of success. In Australia, 53 percent of pregnancies at one major center occurred in the first IVF cycle, 27 percent in the second, 11 percent in the third, and 5 percent or less in the fourth through seventh attempts.[39] Women who are "poor responders" and do not respond to medication are unlikely to conceive in repeated attempts. Moreover, poor responders yielded fewer eggs on average. Their response was even lower if they only had one ovary.[40]

Other studies have shown IVF is only marginally successfully for women with idiopathic infertility or severe endometriosis.[41] Its success is mixed when the male partner has a low sperm count. It is most effective for tubal infertility and it is expected to help an estimated 80 percent of women with tubal blockages. In vitro fertilization is "clearly applicable" only in 18 percent of all infertility, according to one British study, although it is thought to be the only hope for women with tubal infertility.[42]

In summary, only with this kind of information can women exercise autonomy and participate in decisions about IVF. The global 20 percent figure fails to take into account that one can arrive at a rough assessment of the odds of success for any particular woman. For example, a person who has virtually no chance of success would have the following traits:

- over 40 years old
- at a new center with no births
- several unsuccessful attempts at ovulation induction
- husband with low sperm count
- unsuccessful IVF attempts
- severe endometriosis

A woman with a good chance of success would have the following traits:

- between 25 and 34 years old
- at an established center with multiple births
- only one or two unsuccessful IVF attempts
- husband with high sperm count
- tubal infertility with no other problems

Only the patient can ultimately make this calculation. For all the physician's good intentions, including the often held assumption that the patient does not want to be overwhelmed with information, it is imperative that physicians give and patients ask for as detailed an account as possible. Otherwise the gambling mentality can too easily take hold, with women, convinced the next roll of the dice will do the trick, developing strategies of either going from center to center (changing the slot machines) or staying at the same center until or if the center refuses to continue trying. One woman expressed the seduction of IVF: "I couldn't decide not to try it. You can put too much energy into it. The more you try, the more important it gets. I'm worried about losing perspective. It [IVF] is more important now because I didn't get pregnant [after the first attempt]. I just got more determined."

ASSUMING RESPONSIBILITY

Taking on the role of a discriminating consumer of basic and expanded IVF is a hard task in a society that deifies technology, praises "gutsiness," and projects misleading symbols. Instead, it is easier to hand decision making to the seduction of modern technology, as did the woman who averred: "At twenty-six, I adamantly refused to give up hope that some miracle—either at the hand of modern medicine or left to nature—would defy those unbeatable odds while I was still in my childbearing years."

An important question in the beginning of the era of expanded IVF is

71

to ask to what extent the patient ought to assume responsibility for the "goodness" of the way IVF is offered. If the patient is viewed as a vulnerable supplicant, not much can be expected of her as a reformer. Moreover, some patients, as in all medical fields, prefer a paternalistic model of interaction with physicians, have no interest in reviewing statistics, and are more interested in securing their personal goal of motherhood than making political statements. For those burdened with the struggle of infertility and for those deferential to physicians in any case, paternalism may be the model of choice. This patient asks minimal questions, is uninclined to challenge physicians, and is unlikely to speak publicly against any feature of IVF.

Other patients, however, can take on a mantle of discriminating consumption without jeopardizing (and probably enhancing) their primary goal of having a baby. It is not unreasonable or an example of "blaming the victim" to suggest that patients ought to take on greater responsibility as models of discriminating consumption of IVF. These patients will assume roles as a knowledgeable consumer, negotiator, and citizen of a technological age. As a consumer, she will ask pointed questions of the practitioners. She will want to know the number of births at the center in which she is interested, will get a breakdown of who succeeded and who did not, a detailed track record of the percent of patients who go to laparoscopy, the percent of time eggs are retrieved, and the percent of time they fertilize not only for IVF in general, but for IVF as practiced at that center. She will accept as bona fide only those pregnancy rates based on fetal heartbeats. She will ask the same questions of success rates for IVF's variations, such as embryo freezing, both at all centers and at that particular center. If no successes have occurred, it is appropriate for her to ask for reduced financial charges.

The patient as consumer will ask questions. Physicians themselves express surprise at how few questions many patients ask (and mean). They suggest finding a center with births, qualified staff including certified endocrinolgists and embryologists who have worked with human embryos; and persons in the laboratory who have had successes, either at that center or at another. The patient will want access to counseling, if necessary. First-time patients will ask to speak with former patients on the telephone before trying. If they need to interact with other couples, they should find out how many patients go through IVF at any one time. They should be assured someone will be available to answer questions at odd times, on weekends, and in evenings.

The responsible patient will act as a negotiator by going into a center with a pre-set idea of how much she is willing to invest in the procedure.

It is less responsible to "try as often as it takes"; this does not take into account the many factors that affect success rates. The high rate of miscarriages among women who get pregnant from IVF and who are over forty years old, for example, might be enough to dissuade those women from trying it as often as it takes. Here an alternative resolution, such as learning more about infertility from the IVF experience, might be more appropriate and help ease the disappointment of fashioning a lower expectation of success.

Patients will be public spirited if they avoid asking more of reproductive techniques than they can give. This means resisting the urge to deify IVF. Pure grit is not enough to produce a baby in the face of stubborn physically based infertility; at some point technology cannot help. The patient will resist participating in the fiction that IVF babies are miracle babies; IVF is an earthly invention, complete with flaws.

The discriminating patient will be careful about the images of desperation and their implications for the status of women. Desperation perpetuates myths of irrational, emotional decision making, sets women up as potential victims, and pushes an idea of the motherhood imperative. The discriminating patient will search for authentic reasons for trying IVF in order to avoid becoming a victim of needs created by the presence of sophisticated techniques.

If a model of autonomy is championed by some IVF patients who communicate it to physicians, other patients, and the public by telling their stories, such women blaze a path of circumspect consumption that will give guidance as our society faces expanded IVF. Patients vary widely in their backgrounds, ability to set limits, and the expectations they hold for IVF. It makes sense to assume that those willing to assert limits speak out and help reshape the stereotype that depicts them as relentless consumers of the new reproductive techniques. In doing so they send messages about other new techniques as well. Perri Klass, a physician who was pregnant while in medical school, tells of an exchange with a fellow student who asked if she were going to have amniocentesis, a test done on pregnant women to determine if the fetus has abnormalities, such as sickle-cell anemia, which is a disease limited almost exclusively to blacks:

The climax came when a young man in my class asked me, "Have you had all those genetic tests? Like for sickle-cell anemia?"

I looked at him. He is white. I am white. "I'm not in the risk group for sickle-cell," I said gently.

73

"Yeah, I know," he said, "but if there's even a one-in-a-zillion chance—.[43]

The "one-in-a-zillion" mentality, tailored to the western ethos that pins hope on technology, creates needs that individuals did not even know they had. The creation of needs knows no boundaries and will predictably increase in the era of expanded IVF, with its tests for genetic abnormalities and possibilities for assorted life-style choices. The time to question indiscriminate consumption is now, before patterns of behavior are set. Scientists, physicians, and the public in general press toward expanding consumption. Ultimately, however, the responsibility for circumspect consumption must be shared by patients themselves.

CHAPTER FIVE

A Responsible Government

The attention our society has given to IVF signals our reluctance to give carte blanche power to physicians to monitor IVF.[1] We face a bind, however, over how much governmental involvement we want in the intimate matter of childbearing. On the one hand, we see procreation as a private matter and we distrust efforts by the government to monitor conception.[2] On the other hand, some among us fume about governmental inaction in the area of IVF. Among other things, observers claim that letting new conceptions go ahead without oversight would be "disastrous," the states have done "nothing very useful" in the new reproduction area, the U.S. political effort amounts to an "embarrassing history" in comparison with other western democracies, and the federal government is guilty of "stark irresponsibility" in not funding IVF research and in losing an avenue for monitoring research in the process.[3] Should the government lend its weight to a matter with an exquisitely private foundation? Or should the authority largely be enjoyed by patients and physicians?

This chapter looks at efforts by both the private sector (physicians) and public sector (state and national governments) to monitor IVF. It argues that governmental action to this point has reflected misguided intentions and that policy can and should develop only when our knowledge of public values is better understood and respected. It calls for an approach of gradual and delayed policy, while in the meantime the government encourages an understanding of public values about reproductive techniques. The chapter begins with a look at the federal government's early reaction to IVF which set a pattern of inauthenticity that today can be undone only by deliberate action.

THE FEDERAL GOVERNMENT AND IVF

The federal government, painted in fiction as the ugly intruder into reproduction—the Big Brother and destroyer of initiative—is in the area of new conceptions, the meekest of actors. Politicians have hitched up their trousers and tiptoed away from the IVF issue. Because IVF is set in a constitutional context of procreational privacy, this inaction may well be to the advantage of IVF. The problem, however, is that politicians have left the scene for reasons having little to do with the substantive merits of new conceptions. Irresponsibility comes from having made decisions on the basis of tangential issues rather than confronting the issues of IVF that warrant examination in their own right.

The government's response to IVF can be told through one of the persons, along with Doris Del Zio, Landrum Shettles, Robert Edwards, Paul Ramsey, and Lesley Brown who, we can see with hindsight, was an early actor through whom patterns of IVF became set. In this case the person was Pierre Soupart, a professor of gynecology at Vanderbilt University who, in 1977, mailed a 57-page, single-spaced research proposal to the federal government. The proposal, filled with the language of cytogenetic analysis, aneuploidy, blastomeres, meiosis, and oocyte maturation,[4] pitched the subject of human IVF into the political field. It prompted an unexpected volley with retorts that echo to this day.

In the 1970s IVF was a scientist's dream: elegantly simple and filled with promises of practical applications and answers to theoretical questions about the origin of life. In the 1970s IVF was a policymaker's nemesis: little understood, born into the legacy of the fictional Brave New World, and posing a cornucopia of regulatory challenges. James Watson had painted a bleak picture of IVF in Congressional testimony in 1971 and had issued the same warnings in the pages of *Atlantic Monthly*, the best-selling book *Future Shock* predicted cloning just around the corner, and a prominent sociologist predicted somber consequences of IVF which would include gender maldistribution and an increase in crime.[5]

In 1973 the U.S. Supreme Court legalized abortion,[6] a decision which gave rise to a tenacious group of attentive citizens, organized around the National Right to Life Committee, who, on religious and moral grounds, committed their resources to protecting fetuses. In the wake of their efforts to limit abortion and research on aborted and about-to-be aborted fetuses, the state legislatures passed a series of laws forbidding fetal and/ or embryo research[7] which foretold the strength of the right-to-life lobby.

Wary of what IVF might portend, skittish about the abortion controversy, and aware of efforts by Edwards and Steptoe to fertilize human eggs externally, federal officials took steps to prepare for the likelihood that researchers would send proposals involving IVF to agencies such as the National Institutes of Health. Over a period of two years, a terse policy was developed in the Department of Health, Education, and Welfare (DHEW).[8] If DHEW received a proposal regarding human IVF research, the Secretary would appoint a board to review IVF for its ethical acceptability.

No application or proposal involving human *in vitro* fertilization may be funded by the Department or any component thereof until the application or proposal has been reviewed by the Ethical Advisory Board and the Board has rendered advice as to its acceptability from an ethical standpoint.[9]

Thus, IVF took on the mantle of an ethical issue. Research on human embryos was to pass ethical as well as scientific muster.

Pierre Soupart was aware that Edwards and Steptoe were transferring externally fertilized embryos to women in the hope of obtaining a pregnancy. He preferred, however, to study the safety of IVF before actually transferring embryos to the uteruses of women. For this purpose he proposed to take eggs from women undergoing sterilization,[10] fertilize them in vitro, and study the fertilized eggs for chromosomal abnormalities. He planned to discard the embryos rather than transfer them to women for possible pregnancies. Soupart's university approved the proposal through traditional avenues of review and through a special ethics committee convened because of the sensitivity of IVF. Soupart's motives were several. According to a colleague at Vanderbilt: "He was preoccupied with learning about the reproductive process. He wanted to help people have a child. Also, more importantly, he had the scientist's hunger to know how this all works. He was in awe of it."

The National Institutes of Health, the agency to which Soupart submitted the proposal "Cytogenetics of Human Preimplantation Embryos," approved Soupart's proposal for funding in October 1977.[11] "Still, the mandated Ethics Advisory Board (EAB) had to be set up to review the proposal. This put a wedge in Soupart's timing but not, he thought, a significant one. "Expecting prompt approval" of his proposal, he found instead that months later no EAB had been set up. The months and years that passed may not have been long in the world of the bureaucrat but they were deathly long to Soupart, who had virtually suspended his project for three years due to these political "circumstances totally out of our control."[12] As Soupart waited for the EAB to be set up, he learned of the first ongoing pregnancy in Britain of a fetus fertilized externally.

If Soupart and other potential IVF practitioners were distressed about footdragging at DHEW, their concern may have been lessened by the EAB members eventually selected. They made up a staid group of eleven men and two women; seven physicians, one attorney, two medical ethicists, three persons involved in public affairs, and two adjunct consultants (an attorney and an ethicist).[13]

The Secretary of DHEW, Joseph Califano, sent a letter of direction to the EAB two months after Louise Brown's birth. In vitro fertilization surely promised benefits for infertile couples, he wrote, but the EAB was to weigh these benefits against the costs IVF might bring. In vitro fertilization raised a "panoply" of "serious moral and ethical questions" that were "complex and sensitive," and "extraordinarily difficult," he wrote, and they "reach[ed] to our most profound moral and ethical beliefs." Moreover, it was not clear what would happen *next:*

Can techniques of *in vitro* fertilization and transplantation of the embryo damage the resulting fetus and lead to abnormal children? Will this research lead to selective breeding, to attempts to control the genetic makeup of offspring or to the use of "surrogate parents," where, for example, rich women might pay poor women to carry their children?[14]

The EAB members, Califano wrote, were to "conduct a thorough examination" of the issues, "solicit the widest possible public comment on these questions," "consult thoroughly with ethicists and social and political representatives," and assure "wide public dissemination" of the results.

Two lines of thinking appeared in the two documents on Califano's desk. Soupart's proposal framed the matter in scientific terms with a specific intention of testing the safety of a medical technique for dealing with tubal infertility. In it, an individual ethic and presumption of benefit prevailed. Califano's letter framed the matter as a broad issue with questions of social accountability. In it, a social ethic and presumption of possible dysfunctionality prevailed.

The EAB met in eleven cities across the country,[15] and gathered oral testimony from 179 people, written testimony from eighteen others, and

2,000 items from interest groups and other citizens. This was a time when most of the public supported IVF, as indicated by opinion polls.[16] This same presumption of benefit, which was captured in Soupart's proposal, also carried through in the EAB report, which appeared in the *Federal Register* in June 1979.[17]

Diplomacy permeated the report, which had about it the restrained tone of a commission document.[18] The report concluded that the technique was ethically acceptable for married couples and that research on human embryos was acceptable when the research was designed to establish IVF safety, the question would yield "important scientific information," the method complied with federal laws governing research on human subjects, tissue donors gave informed consent, and the embryos were not kept alive for more than fourteen days after fertilization.[19] Researchers were obligated to inform the public if the studies showed IVF endangered unborn offspring.

The report's central presumption was that IVF was intimately connected with the couple's "personal and marital privacy" to make reproductive choices. Its tone advised against governmental regulation; on the contrary, one must "guard against unwarranted governmental intrusion" in matters of reproductive choice. The government could restrict reproductive autonomy but only for a "compelling state interest" such as "protecting the health and safety of mothers and offspring." Interference was not warranted for "uncertain or remote" dangers such as cloning, genetic hybrids, or genetic engineering. Where the "opportunity for abuse" existed, it could be checked when the need arose by legislative action or "good judgment." At present, the government's role was not to prohibit IVF but to educate people so they could make "fully informed choices about reproduction" on their own.

The question of the embryo's status had concerned ethicists, and the EAB addressed it in a way that was to be repeated in the years to come: the "human embryo is entitled to profound respect; but this respect does not necessarily encompass the full legal and moral rights attributed to persons." More important are the interests of actual persons—the couples seeking to reproduce and the scientists prepared to conduct scientific research.

The EAB thought the private and public sectors could share responsibility for IVF. Under this power-sharing model, the government's role would be affirmative; it would fund research proposals, initiate data gathering about IVF from around the world,[20] and encourage states to pass laws defining the rights and responsibilities of the people involved in IVF. The private sector's role would revolve around self-regulation; it would monitor itself through professional organizations and the network of Institutional Review Boards, through which medical peers evaluate research proposals.

How little could Soupart have predicted that with a supportive report such as this behind him, DHEW would drop his proposal like a hot potato?[21] Not only did Soupart not receive the $395,630 for which he asked, but the climate of rejection was so resounding that for the next decade no other researchers even applied for federal funding for IVF studies. Soupart was reportedly "broken" by the experience, and shortly thereafter he was dead, with his death in 1981 from cancer hastened, at least one of his colleagues conjectured, by the delays and frustrations of the experience that had thrust him into a political thicket of the kind that fed medical lore that politicians were not the right persons to make decisions about medical research. The events following the publication of the EAB report gave the first solid indication that IVF was going to be embroiled in an issue not of its own making—the seemingly intractable matter of abortion.

The EAB members had predicted at their last meeting that the report would fan the fires of the abortion debate[22] and they were correct. In the year following the report's publication, DHEW received 12,600 letters from across the country. Most (80 percent) came from individuals; 16 percent were signed by two persons; and 4 percent were signed by three persons or were petitions with many signatures. One organization sent petitions with 25,000 signatures.[23]

Only 2 percent of the letters supported IVF and they did so on the grounds that the procedure would help infertile couples. The rest of the letters opposed IVF, but very few letter writers mentioned the EAB's recommendations. Instead, they wrote that IVF was inherently immoral, the destruction of embryos brought to mind Nazi Germany, and the procedure ignored the rights of the embryo. They likened IVF to abortion and argued that IVF's benefits could not stand up against IVF's affronts to the embryo, family, and society. Those who wrote letters in favor of IVF were thinking of the clinical act of IVF and embryo transfer; those who wrote critical letters were thinking of the implications of laboratory research. The two, according to a report summarizing the letters, were "focusing on different aspects of the issues."[24]

Members of Congress contested the EAB report too. Fifty letters containing the signatures of 20 Senators and 73 Representatives reached DHEW. Of the 36 letters containing positions, all criticized IVF.[25] The writers said IVF treaded on the rights of the embryo, was inherently immoral, had grave societal implications, and needed further guidelines.

Only one of the letters mentioned infertile couples.[26] Twenty called for more discussion.

In vitro fertilization had become a pariah attached to the politically dangerous issue of abortion. The EAB report turned out not to be a starting point for more discussion; on the contrary, it was an ending point for a matter federal officials thought better left untouched. When two Senators asked a newly formed commission on human research to review the EAB report, they were told the commissioners had reviewed the report but did not want to take up "premature or duplicative" topics or "pass judgment one way or the other on the merits of any specific conclusion" in the report.[27]

A staff member on the EAB later remarked that the report was simply "too hot to handle."[28] The Department of HEW dropped the issue with dispatch: Soupart's proposal was denied, though not with an explicit letter; Califano tabled the EAB's recommendations; and the next DHEW Secretary, Patricia Harris, disbanded the EAB altogether, apparently believing IVF was a procedure for a wealthy minority of couples.[29] In vitro fertilization at that time had vocal detractors but not vocal promoters. Not all physicians supported IVF in its early days; in fact, the editors of the *Journal of the American Medical Association* had called for a moratorium on human embryo transfer in 1972.[30] The first IVF center in the United States was still a year away; Louise Brown had only just been born and IVF's safety was still not assured; infertile couples were caught in their own struggle against infertility; and no natural empathy existed in Washington's mainly male and predominantly fertile body of politicians for a technique to help a minority of women conceive.

The EAB's disbanding had the effect of foreclosing federal funding of research connected with the clinical practice of IVF and with any studies using human embryos. None of the EAB's recommendations, such as the suggestion that the government fund data gathering on IVF, was enacted. The EAB report, four years in the making, was, and still is, "conscientiously ignored."[31] In vitro fertilization was caught in the web of fears about abortion and genetic engineering, both of which were unpalatable for public officials.[32]

For a politician, the best way to deal with a political thicket is to do nothing, which is what happened. The Congress and President "have been more than happy to leave unexplored a mine field likely to be as explosive as the abortion and Baby Doe controversies."[33] To back IVF research is to court the ire of political groups. Said one former federal official: "Society is very vindictive and it has an elephantine memory" about researchers who proceed with topics before society is ready to go ahead with them. Uncertainty about policy has not only chilled research on human embryos, but it has discouraged open discussion of that research. When clinicians and scientists are asked whether they plan to conduct research involving human embryos, they demure, citing the history of federal policy, and say such research is "just trouble" and a "headache." Periodically, attempts are made to re-establish the Ethics Advisory Board. Despite cynicism among scientists that the EAB or an equivalent will be set up in the near future, an effort is, at the time of this writing, underway to re-establish the Board.[34]

Political factors predominate in the IVF field where the wish of politicians is to stay clear of the matter. As a result, without exploratory studies in IVF's safety in this country, IVF clinics grew rapidly within a few years after the first American IVF birth. The federal policy had the effect of putting the cart (the clinical application of IVF) before the horse (basic research on IVF). There was irony in the fact that IVF was accepted as a clinical treatment but not as a subject of research. It created an "absurd position" of a "growing acceptance of a clinical therapy which we steadfastly refuse to accept as an allowable subject for research."[35]

As a consequence of the political context of IVF, a gentlemen's agreement (in the literal as well as metaphorical sense in that most politicians and IVF practitioners are men) arose by default in which the medical community would be free to govern its own. Policy on IVF today combines self-regulation by the private sector, existing laws designed to protect subjects of research, and a handful of state laws dealing directly with IVF. The initiative, however, is enjoyed primarily by the private sector, where medical groups fashion guidelines for physicians to decide what to allow and what to limit in the field of reproductive technologies. The values emerging in the private sector are not notably different from those expressed in the EAB report. Unfortunately, this status quo was developed by default rather than by a deliberate policy reached by public office holders. Only recently have Congressional hearings been held in which witnesses have suggested specific ways policymakers can legislate to remedy defects in self-regulation.[36]

SELF-REGULATION BY THE PRIVATE SECTOR

A key advantage of leaving physicians and scientists free to regulate themselves is that they see difficulties of the clinical practice of IVF that outsiders are not able to see or are not interested in seeing. To physicians, IVF is a medical craft. They are in a position to see slovenliness in their craft and to know how to remedy it. It is the physician, not the politician, who can see the need for a certified endocrinologist on the staff, for example, or can understand what is required for quality control in the laboratory. If one is looking for reforms that have a direct bearing on the patient, it is the doctors who can identify trouble spots in the medical protocol of IVF. One of the first two statements published by the American Fertility Society (AFS) about IVF, for example, was entitled "Minimal Standards for Programs of In Vitro Fertilization."[37] In it the AFS recommended, among other things, minimum personnel requirements for IVF programs.

Another advantage of self-regulation is that the medical perspective directs attention to matters of quality control that are relatively accessible to reform. This interest in specific features of clinical practice balances the tendency of politicians to define broad "issues" surrounding IVF that are not easily amenable to reform. When physicians recommend personnel standards and minimum standards of care in the laboratory, they help build a record of reforms that in turn enhances public confidence in society's ability to put limits on rapidly changing techniques. Although this inductive record must at some point be combined with attention to the broader implications of alternative conception, the inductive method of problem-solving in the private sector conveys a message of competence and the ability to take deliberate action.

One incentive for self-regulation is the practitioners' distrust of regulation by politicians. Physicians see politicians as interlopers interfering with something outside their expertise. They therefore have an interest in monitoring their own activities in order to stave off what they see as governmental intrusion:

"The government has to stay out of [IVF regulation]. Group consciousness develops in hospitals. The government is not familiar with it."

"In the scientific area, the politicians are not the right persons to be regulating. ... This is uncharted water. ... Government involvement will severely restrict progress."

"There is absolutely no business for the government to be in there. It is just a medical issue. The government is meddling."

A second incentive for self-vigilance is the threat of lawsuits by unhappy patients or persons acting on behalf of children born with problems as a result of new conceptions. The physician's "healthy respect for —or fear of—our tort and malpractice laws" is a long-standing medical incentive to carry out techniques with care and integrity.[38] One IVF practitioner expressed in 1984 his "healthy respect" for lawsuits this way:

> "We haven't had a lawsuit yet. . . . None of the [then] 200 American in vitro babies has had abnormalities. As soon as we get one— watch out. There's gold in them thar hills. They're waiting for us to fall."

The threat of lawsuits sends physicians to hospital attorneys to approve new protocols and consent forms. The lawsuit is a tactical method in which patients as consumers can strike where action is needed. It is like a laser beam that cauterizes a leaking vein, negating the need for general surgery. The lawsuit, regardless of its outcome, identifies and publicizes a problem. The case of the orphaned embryos in Australia pointed to an unanticipated problem in embryo freezing about who was responsible for frozen embryos in the event their progenitors died. As a result of that case, hospitals began asking couples to state what should be done with their embryos in the event of death or divorce. The Baby M case of surrogate motherhood publicized the question of who should have parental rights if a surrogate changed her mind about giving the baby to a contracting couple (see chapter 6).[39]

As a result of court decisions in that case, some surrogacy brokers changed the wording of their contracts, and state legislators studied with new interest ways of regulating the practice.

Judicial decisions provide a context for the gradual accretion of policy. They allow experimentation because the decisions of the individual cases technically obligate only the persons in the jurisdiction in which the decision is handed down. The nonbinding dicta of the appellate court's written opinion let judges grapple with and explore various dimensions of the issue. Legal decisions deal with actual, not hypothetical, injuries, which helps publicize matters of interest to consumers. In the area of surrogate motherhood, for example, unexpected injuries have occurred, including cases in which a baby was born with severe defects, a surrogate died of heart failure late in her pregnancy, and a baby was born with AIDS to a surrogate.[40] If such cases were to become the subject of lawsuits, the added publicity would warn prospective parties to surrogacy of the range of injuries that can occur.

Lawsuits as incentives for medical self-regulation have the disadvantage of burdening couples already weighted down by the financial and

emotional demands
to expect them to at
have already spent larg
disappointment from th
More often couples feel l
feeling vindictive. Only in
out about negative experienc

Another drawback of lawsu
general lack of tangible injuri
born after IVF are of such a ran
IVF as the cause. In 1986, for exa
of the following congenital defects
cended testicle, spina bifida, imperfo
atresia, Dandy Walker syndrome, hy
pupil, and encephalocele.[42] So far, it
abnormalities is not significantly higher
rally, although there are some suggestio
incidence of low birth weights.[43] It is also d
effect relationships between IVF and injuries

Lawsuits have other disadvantages. They ta
are retrospective rather than anticipatory; they
well-being of a society that seems increasingly
resolve its difficulties; and they further frighten
medical field of obstetrics, where malpractice clain
with.

A third incentive for self-regulation, in addition to a
government regulation and to avoid lawsuits, is the inte.
patients. With numerous IVF clinics now in operation,
increasingly selective about where they try IVF. Prospe
contact the American Fertility Society for a list of centers c
Some couples send, with the aid of word processors, letters to
find out and compare procedures, success rates, and costs. Othe
share experiences about IVF centers in infertility support group
ters with minimal success surely lose referrals from physicians
sending their patients to an unsuccessful center.

The marketplace is, however, an incomplete and sometimes un
mechanism. As IVF becomes more like a business, with chains a
marketing strategies, good but small centers may be swept out becaus
of nonaggressive advertising. Private clinics, which can advertise, pose
sometimes lethal competition for university-based clinics which cannot
advertise. In addition, not all couples have the incentive, resources, or

shop among centers and travel to the most successful of

ntrol in the IVF field comes largely from the weight of the
self. Few persons have a greater interest in making sure
"monster births" than the doctors whose business depends
id reputation of the IVF procedure. Given the mercurial
VF's acceptance by society, IVF practitioners have an interest
negative publicity to a minimum. The elite of the IVF com-
ncluding the first generation clinic founders, are among the
n the effort to introduce quality control through norms that
e on professional status, pride, and competition.

such effort is the formation of a special interest group—a kind
Beta Kappa of IVF practitioners—within the American Fertility
y (AFS) that uses selective membership to create a set of practi-
s whose membership in the group signals quality. The group,
nally known as the IVF Special Interest Group, but now the Society
ssisted Reproductive Technology (SART), was formed in 1984.
ectors of IVF clinics apply for membership and are accepted if their
grams meet minimum standards. Member programs must perform
rty or more IVF cycles each year, have had three or more births, and
eet personnel standards.[45]

Another effort is the American Fertility Society's formation in 1986
of a Registry for collecting and monitoring data from IVF programs. The
Registry gathers data from SART member programs on the number of
patients, IVF cycles started, embryo transfers, clinical pregnancies, abnormal births, and information about related techniques such as GIFT,
donor eggs, and frozen embryos.[46] The AFS compiles a list of programs
meeting the criteria for SART membership[47] and sends this short list to
prospective patients.

Using professional status to bring about quality control appeals to
competitive instincts among physicians. When asked about challenges
facing IVF in the next five years, practitioners refer to the need to keep
"every Tom, Dick, and Harry *off* the bandwagon," "restricting it to
successful centers," "hav[ing] IVF done by people who know what they
are doing," and "standardizing and reviewing of all programs and statistics."[48] Whether to protect their own patient roster or to promote IVF's
image as a respectable field, physicians have taken specific steps to
monitor who practices IVF.

Self-regulation places the IVF elite at the helm, which may or may
not be in the society's best interest, depending on the values held by the
elite. It is not unreasonable to suppose that as time passes, the elite will

shift from the clinicians to research-oriented scientists for whom IVF is not an end in itself but a means to greater knowledge of reproduction and genetics. The "goodness" of IVF self-regulation through internal competition depends upon whether the values of the IVF elite mirror those expressed in the public debate.

Professional norms appear in guidelines published by the AFS and the American College of Obstetricians and Gynecologists (ACOG). Each group has committees that make recommendations about administering IVF. The director of the first American IVF clinic, Howard W. Jones, Jr., said "We don't believe there are any [IVF centers] operating under suboptimal conditions, but [we] are putting forth standards as a precautionary measure" in reference to the recommendations in 1984 of the AFS regarding minimum personnel requirements and other measures to ensure quality control at IVF centers.[49]

Guidelines also help physicians weigh what limits, if any, physicians should place on the choices offered by reproductive technologies. Ethical standards published by the AFS and ACOG in 1984 and 1986 are not unlike political party platforms inasmuch as they convey a sense of direction to practitioners. Like a platform, they capsulize a reasonably coherent belief system about the perceived place of reproductive technologies in society. Whether one agrees or not with the substance of the belief system, the guidelines act as a mechanism around which discussion can be generated. In addition, ethicists and other nonmedical people sometimes sit on the committees, which means the recommendations represent a cross-disciplinary consensus.[50]

A weakness of guidelines is that, as noted in chapter 3, very few practitioners read them carefully. In addition, at least one director has suggested that the guidelines are more for people outside the field than for those inside. Committee reports, as documents reached by consensus and meant for general as well as professional readership, are not analytically rigorous nor is their logic developed in great detail.

A group of physicians, ethicists, and lawyers produced the 1986 AFS guidelines, "Ethical Considerations of the New Reproductive Technologies." As a belief system, these private sector guidelines correspond with the basic principles set in the 1979 public sector EAB report. The new conceptions are a service to society that can "help infertile couples and pregnant women," note the authors, and are, on balance, beneficial. According to an ACOG report, their promise is so great that society has a "moral duty" to help couples in need and practitioners have an obligation to "develop new and better methods of providing care to pregnant women, infertile couples, early embryos, and future children."[51]

The AFS guidelines justify reproductive techniques by placing them squarely in the supportive context of the U.S. Constitution. Scientists enjoy a freedom of inquiry unfettered by public regulation, and married couples have a "right to reproduce" and to select from the choices offered by laboratory conception. Couples enjoy a "liberty" of procreation, grounded in Supreme Court doctrine, and have the right to make choices governed largely by their own consciences: "Infertile couples should, freely and according to the dictate of their own conscience and moral belief, decide whether they wish to avail themselves of the newer technological advances in the field of reproduction."[52]

The guidelines suggest as a method of evaluating new conceptions a cost/benefit rationale in which the costs of each technique are weighed against their benefits. If the benefits outweigh the costs, the technique is ethically permissible. The committee members weighed the costs and benefits of several new conceptions: ovum transfer; sperm, egg, and embryo donation; surrogate motherhood; and surrogate gestational motherhood. Their framework was simple: they asked for each, what are the risks? what are the benefits? do the benefits outweigh the risks?

For the most part, the members concluded that benefits outweighed risks, although they advised caution about untested techniques or those opening so many social and legal conundrums that they would divert doctors from the primary goal of providing medical care to patients. They were cautious about unlimited applications of expanded IVF. Embryo donation, for example, is acceptable only when both wife and husband are medically infertile. It should not be done for convenience, cosmetics, or to produce a "superbaby."[53]

The committee members were not radical pioneers, but neither were they nervous conservatives. Instead, they conveyed a middle-range message of trusting optimism that practitioners could draw the line at common sense and that expanded IVF offered benefits for patients and society. They also conveyed this belief about embryo research, which is a more sensitive issue than clinical IVF. Research using human embryos will advance success rates in IVF and act as a stepping stone for future discoveries.[54] It is permissible, the members felt, for embryos to be created for study in order to achieve more valid findings than with studies using embryos left over from IVF.[55] The researcher bears the burden of showing the worthiness of any study using embryos, and the research should provide a "significant and recognizable potential for generating important new knowledge—not otherwise obtainable—for benefitting human health." The research question must be important enough (the benefit) to justify using human embryos (the cost). It must need human (as opposed to animal) embryos, use the smallest number of embryos possible, and not put the egg donor at risk,[56] and be framed with the aid of Institutional Review Boards and, perhaps, with special consultants. "At this time," wrote the members, it is appropriate to keep embryos alive for fourteen days only.

While urging restraint, the guidelines leave the door open for liberal research: "Such a conservative posture [about embryo research] ... should not preclude truly innovative research directed toward important scientific or clinical advances."[57] This permissive message, repeated in the final paragraph of the report, brings to mind a person advising a friend how to avoid a scuffle: "Keep calm, count to ten, turn the other cheek. If you do fight, however, be sure to win." Caution is advisable. In the face of exciting research, however, scientists can appropriately pursue the knowledge.

One practitioner of IVF in this country thinks that "medicine in general has done very well in this matter by regulating itself."[58] The AFS believes that without a central government mechanism, the organization can take an active role in educating and training IVF practitioners and regulating the enterprise.[59] The AFS is ready to help the medical community "promote," "initiate," and "encourage" the management of reproductive technologies. The gentlemen's agreement works in fine order in the minds of IVF's practitioners, who claim for themselves the right to manage new conceptions according to their judgment, medical expertise, and awareness of effective ways of asserting peer pressure.

The medical sector initiative counterbalances the government's early reactions to IVF. In the Soupart years several messages emerged from the government's reaction: IVF is inherently problematic, it raises issues on a par with abortion, grave problems inhere in its future implications for society, and the debate ought to revolve around the symbolic and moral worth of the human embryo.

The private sector, through self-policing activities and public statements, has sent a message different in nearly every respect: IVF is a service, it is a matter to be considered on its own merits apart from issues such as abortion, the problems inhere in quality control for the clinical application of IVF, and the debate ought to revolve around service to and options for the patients. The embryo is to be treated with respect, but it is not a human. Reproductive technologies ought to be approached with a case by case, inductive, and individualistic frame of mind. Privacy, autonomy, and liberty are the starting points for individual rights,[60] discretion,[61] and ownership.[62] With initiative in the hands of the private sector, IVF has been defined as a medical and private matter.

The private sector has put limits on IVF protocol more effectively than the public sector. Its methods are largely voluntary. The belief system feeds an ideology of individual choice and presumed service to society from basic and expanded IVF. Yet it promotes a belief in what might be called accordian consumption in which a folded fan of applications exists. As societal norms change and knowledge is gained, the fan slowly opens. Physicians have taken steps toward self-regulation but their activities suggest that they will not rigorously question the values underlying new conceptions. We must look elsewhere for a serious debate of the limits we ought to place on the potentially voluminous unfolding fan. In the meantime, the private sector bears a responsibility for continuing to find ways to police the clinical practice of basic and expanded IVF.

REGULATION BY THE PUBLIC SECTOR

I rrespective of the smooth functioning of the gentlemen's agreement, pressures for change exist. Publicly expressed concerns about the techniques are irrepressible, especially with new variations, and scientists and laypersons alike doubt the private sector can or ought to continue its mantle of leadership. Moreover, the inability or unwillingness of policymakers to present reasoned policy alternatives raises questions of their competence and sends a worrisome message to the public about the ability of their governors to handle issues in a technological era.

This is a society in which the public expects policymakers to "do something" in the face of a challenge. In 1984 Congress stepped into the field of IVF when a subcommittee of the House Committee on Science and Technology held one and one-half days of hearings on human embryo transfer. The subcommittee chair, Albert Gore, Jr., introduced the hearings with the battle-ready language of one keen on "doing something" about the new reproductive technologies. The subcommittee had to "grapple" and "wrestle" with IVF, he said. In vitro fertilization raises "sensitive" and "difficult" issues, "challenges" our traditional ideas about parenthood and adoption, and "forces" us to reassess our legal and ethical ways of looking at things.[63]

In the hearings, during which witnesses chided the government for the "embarrassing history" of the Americans in responding to the new techniques compared with records in other western democracies, one witness encapsulated the "do something" ethic with his observation that: "Just because we can't answer all the questions, and we can't, doesn't mean we shouldn't start answering the ones we can answer."[64] Within the overall umbrella of state and national government, then, there are persistent questions about what policymakers should do, motivated by the assumption that the governors must do something. The word government comes from the Latin *gubernare*—to steer—and it is precisely that which critical observers expect public officials to do in relation to reproductive technologies.

If the government is designed to steer, the American policy system provides a number of wheels and drivers for the task. The U.S. government is like a many headed hydra with its endless points of access into policymaking. Will it be federal action? state action? local action? Will it be executive, legislative, or judicial action? Will it be a centralized and direct law passed by the federal legislature? Or will it be decentralized and indirect, such as the existing system of Institutional Review Boards that review proposals for research? The policy with a great impact on IVF—the requirement of the mid-1970s that proposals must pass through an EAB—was a nondescript executive policy enacted by appointed decision makers. The wealth of choice is at the heart of American pluralism. A key matter about IVF policy is to ask, "by whom?"

It is also necessary to ask about policy, "what shall it be?" Policy can variously forbid, regulate, aid, or ignore an activity. What should the prominent ethic in the field of reproductive techniques be? Should the government bar some applications of IVF? Regulate their use? Ease their operation? If the government ventures from its fairly safe position of inaction, should it act primarily in the capacity of prohibitor, regulator, or helper, or should it combine these roles? The sections below look at the merits and drawbacks of three broad approaches to policy: regulatory, affirmative, and deliberate inaction.

REGULATORY POLICY

Outright Prohibitions. To ban or prohibit activities parallels Paul Ramsey's search for the "nevers" and leads us to ask if there are some features of the new technologies so reprehensible that they warrant banning and so antithetical to the sensitivities of Western cultures that it is not enough to trust the private sector to refrain voluntarily from doing them. The authors of the British Warnock report on new reproductive technologies indicated that some agreement on prohibitions is necessary for a well-functioning society: a society with moral scruples is one that imposes "some barriers that are not to be crossed, some limits fixed, beyond which people must not be allowed to go."[65]

Certainly there are applications of laboratory conception that seem inherently distasteful for our values as humans. For example, scientists have crossed a sheep and a goat and ended up with a new species—the geep. Might they one day be able to cross a human and a gorilla and end up with a new species—the guman or horilla? Is the cross-fertilization of human and animal gametes something the government ought to ban?

On the one hand, banning cross-species fertilization would be a comforting indictment against an application that seems to violate the natural law of respect for the integrity of the human being. It gives relief to know we can limit and have limited seemingly undesirable behavior. On the other hand, prohibitions are only incomplete answers in that they penalize activities but do not eliminate the chance the activities will be done anyway. Moreover, a prohibition is a hollow victory if the thing banned has no real chance of coming to fruition. The horilla is simply not on the scientific horizon; it takes few policy skills to ban something that exists in the imagination rather than in fact. By passing laws that anticipate events far in the future, society runs the risk of passing laws that languish, suffer from desuetude, and eventually promote cynicism about superflous legislation.

Banning also rejects the possibility that values will change and that which seems reprehensible will be acceptable in the future. In the 1940s, for example, a censorship board found a Walt Disney film showing the birth of a buffalo obscene;[66] such a decision would be anathema to today's standards. Banning also runs counter to basic optimism in our society by presuming all applications of a technique are equally negative. In fact, some applications may be beneficial. A flat ban on all cross-species fertilizations would take within its sweep the 'humster" test for assessing the penetrability of male sperm. With this test, human sperm are mixed with hamster eggs. The resulting hybrid cannot live beyond a small number of cells and can never grow into an actual humster. The ban would not further the intention of preventing new species; moreover, it would eliminate legitimate activities. The ban would impose a cost (lost knowledge) without a corresponding benefit.

Banning activities in their entirety conveys a message of distrust about scientists and technicians. As one embryologist said about distasteful applications, "people have to remember that we are humans too." To ban something projected in the future is to give voice to the technological imperative that what can happen will happen, it reinforces fears of the general public, and it feeds sensationalism. In Victoria, Australia, legislators hastily passed a law banning cloning without clearly defining cloning. In so doing it fed the idea that cloning is a near possibility but did nothing to allay public fears about what cloning is.[67] The ambiguity has necessitated repeated clarifications of the law.[68]

Finally, prohibiting scientific endeavors runs contrary to our history offering constitutional protection to research and inquiry.[69] Recent efforts by the federal government to bar recombinant DNA research represent a new dimension of governmental activity. Prohibitions on research are acceptable only for the most compelling reasons. Prohibitions are best if drawn narrowly to avoid taking legitimate behaviors within their sweep. The British Warnock commission, for example, recommended that cross-species fertilizations using human gametes be forbidden only beyond the two-cell stage.[70] This narrowly crafted prohibition would not forbid the humster test as a diagnostic tool in infertility. Its model is preferable to a broad-ranging ban.

Outright prohibitions ought to be done only under commonly accepted and rigorous standards similar to those used by the courts in interpreting the constitution. Among the tests might be a "compelling state interest," "assault on sensibilities," or "inherently reprehensible" test. The judicial standards of proximity and degree are appropriate. Activities will be barred only if they are proximate (clear and present) and inherently dangerous (degree) to a compelling state interest.[71]

Regulations. An alternative to outright prohibitions is the regulation of the time, place, and manner of activities thought to be in need of oversight. In Britain, for example, a Voluntary Licensing Authority (VLA) monitors IVF centers conducting research using human embryos. The VLA is made up of lay members and members of the Medical Research Council and Royal College of Obstetricians and Gynaecologists,[72] and it gathers information from visits to research centers. At present, it will not approve four kinds of research: modifying a human embryo's genetic composition, placing a human embryo in another species for gestation, cloning an embryo, or growing an embryo for more than fourteen days.[73] Members of Parliament have proposed changing this voluntary agency into a state-backed agency, the Statutory Licensing Authority.[74]

By not approving certain kinds of research, the VLA (or SLA) regulates research but does not formally ban it. To illustrate, in 1986 it requested one center to show it had a policy for disposing of spare embryos, and in that year the VLA approved licensing for all but one center.[75]

Given the drawbacks of prohibitions on research and practice as described above, it is reasonable to suggest that regulation is preferable to banning. This leads to the question of the level of government that ought to do the regulating. Much of the critics' anger about IVF policy is directed toward the federal government, which has been reticent about directing policy debate or setting up a forum for discussing the issues. Federal involvement has a number of advantages. It creates a reasonably centralized forum for discussing reproductive techniques in that matters debated within Congress draw national attention in a way that debates within state legislatures cannot. Congressional hearings draw witnesses from across the country and efficiently marshal timely data about an issue. Testimony at the committee hearings is published and available for public reading in repository libraries. Bills introduced to Congress label a matter an issue with national implications and legitimize it by sending the message that the matter is worthy of review.

A drawback of Congressional involvement is that federal legislators appear to have trouble discussing IVF as an issue on its own merits. The controversial issue of abortion and the political fears it raises stubbornly cloak questions of the substantive merits of the new conceptions. Even the Congressional Biomedical Ethics Board, passed in 1985 and seemingly a neutral review agency, has encountered early troubles because the abortion issue has left it "endlessly bogged down in politics" as legislators tried to balance its membership with "pro-life" supporters.[76] Some Senators introduced bills in Congress to provide child adoption benefits for federal government employees *except* for children conceived through IVF, donor insemination, or surrogate motherhood, which seems deliberately to penalize new conceptions.[77] The lingering inauthenticity in federal involvement in IVF suggests that regulations might still be premature, although steps toward more dispassionate inquiry continue to be taken.[78] It does not benefit society when policy parading as policy of the new conceptions is, in reality, part of the lingering controversy over abortion.

Another drawback of Congressional action is that the federal government has historically not been involved in medical regulation. Instead, writes Gary B. Ellis of the Office of Technology Assessment, in the medical field "quality assurance and consumer protection issues are left to State legislatures, professional societies, consumer groups, and word-of-mouth." The Food and Drug Administration tests and monitors "drugs and devices" and Congress oversees matters in Veterans' Administration hospitals but aside from these and other types of broad jurisdiction, the federal government is little involved in oversight of medical practice.[79] It would be highly unusual for Congress to set up licensing criteria for IVF facilities, for example, or take other action directly affecting the daily operation of IVF clinics. Such action would be a matter more normally left to the states.

The state legislatures have played a limited but visible role in the evolving policy of IVF. As policymakers, states are often relegated to the role of "whipping posts of commentators who believe things should be better."[80] In fact, however, the states, with their differing history, culture, economy, and legacy of morality, can act as laboratories for the development of complex policy where there is little national consensus. The diverse policy that some see as a weakness of state government is a strength if one is looking for creative solutions to technological problems.

Over the years, the states have banned the death penalty, reduced speed limits, and imposed pollution control standards for automobiles before the national government took action. They also operate programs in areas that seem outside the purview of the national government, such as water sanitation programs, monitoring of restaurants, and oversight of higher education. They have taken on the role of an experimental laboratory for the development of policy.[81] This role is appropriate in the field of alternative conception, where the federal government is stymied and where coherent national policy may be still impossible to implement.

Experimentation in state legislatures can be done with bounded impacts. For example, if surrogate motherhood is regulated in one state, other states can learn from the impact of the law's provisions. Mistakes are confined to the pioneering state; judicial review of the law indicates how its wording or intent can be clarified, and this allows trial and error on a small scale. States have the tendency to model themselves after one another in what is known as a "diffusion of innovations." With this some states (normally those that are populated, wealthy, and urban) act as national or regional leaders in legislation. Follower states in the region or nation then draft their legislation after the model presented by the innovator states.[82] State-by-state modeling helps nationalize a policy and encourage an evolving consensus in the absence of federal legislation.

By looking to innovator states, the follower states have something on which to base their attempts at framing new laws. In addition, model state laws drafted by such agencies as the National Conference of Commissioners on Uniform States Laws [NCCUSL] are available for states to follow. The NCCUSL, for example, has worked on a model law based on state adoption codes to help states interested in protecting the children born from alternative conception.[83] States can also use as a starting point for legislative reforms their existing statutes. To illustrate, states can amend their donor insemination (DI) laws to meet the needs posed by the recent start of egg and embryo donation. Donor insemination laws generally state that the husband who gives consent for artificial insemination is presumed to be the natural father of any child born from DI. This can be amended to state that the wife who gives birth to a baby conceived with a donor egg is presumed to be the natural mother.

A disadvantage of state laws is that their very efficiency can lead to premature or hasty policies that are difficult to uproot once in place. Policy benefits no one if it is instantly outmoded or, worse, found to interfere with the values it was intended to protect. In Massachusetts, a fetal research law seeming to bar IVF was challenged, and the attorney general for the Boston region interpreted the law to mean that all embryos must be transferred to the woman in IVF in order to preserve them.[84] The effect might have been opposite that intended, however, because later data indicated that when too many embryos are transferred at once, implantation rates decline. This produces the ironic situation of policy designed to protect embryos instead endangering them. The Louisiana legislature recently passed a bill defining the embryo as a "juridical person" with the capacity to sue and be sued.[85] The effect is to discourage doctors from discarding embryos. As a result, one IVF-cryopreservation clinic in the state donates all spare embryos but has confronted a dilemma in that, at least in the first few months of operation, more couples want to donate than receive spare embryos.

It is not unreasonable to conclude that states act with more ease when they rule in matters relating to health and safety than when they venture into social policy. Regulations limiting access to IVF or forbidding embryo research raise constitutional questions about procreational privacy and freedom of inquiry. Regulations monitoring the health and safety of clinical IVF, on the other hand, involve the state in more narrowly based matters, such as requiring IVF to be performed only by trained personnel or requiring the genetic screening of egg or embryo donors.

The track record to date of the states indicates the strengths and weaknesses of their contribution. The states have already regulated assisted conceptions. The states have monitored the practice and legal features of artificial insemination by donor (now called donor insemination or DI). Of the 24 states that regulate DI, 14 specify that a licensed physician (or "authorized person" in New York) perform DI; 12 require records to be kept, sealed, and released only under court order; three specify that the donor has no rights or obligations vis-à-vis the child; and all legitimize the child conceived through DI, either by stating the child is legitimate or by stating the consenting husband is the same under law as the natural father.[86]

By 1988, 27 state legislatures had entertained a total of 73 bills relating to surrogate motherhood. Twenty-five of the bills would have forbidden surrogate motherhood, 26 would regulate it, and 22 would establish panels to study it. Louisiana banned surrogacy, and seven states eventually set up study commissions.[87] Twenty-four states forbid a woman from accepting payment for giving her child for adoption,[88] which monitors surrogacy by limiting the conditions under which brokers can use monetary enticements.

Several states have passed laws dealing with IVF. Pennsylvania requires records to be kept of the names, locations, and sponsors of IVF and of the number of eggs fertilized, used, transferred, and destroyed. Illinois passed a law in 1980 providing that any person who united ovum and sperm outside the human body was "deemed to have the care and custody" of the resulting child and was liable for child abuse.[89] This chilled IVF, mainly because it was unclear when the physician's custody ended. One state representative asked in legislative debate if a doctor or nurse who assisted in IVF could "be somehow called upon years later to pay for an appendectomy for [the resulting] child." The bill's sponsor said, "yes."[90]

As a result of a lawsuit by an Illinois couple, the "care and custody" portion of the law was interpreted to mean the responsibility ended after the embryo's transfer.[91] Earlier, the Attorney General of Illinois and the State's Attorney of Cook County wrote that physicians were within the law if they refrained from "wilfully endangering or injuring the embryo." This left a "legal cloud" over IVF in the state, and the ambiguity of the law put physicians in an uncertain position for implementing IVF's variations such as embryo freezing,[92] at least until the law was reinterpreted.

A number of states regulate research on fetuses and/or embryos. Some of these regulations are "inauthentic" in that they were passed with abortion, not IVF, in mind in the aftermath of the *Roe v. Wade* abortion decision. Designed to restrict research on aborted or about-to-be aborted fetuses,[93] their wording gives little clue as to whether preimplantation embryos are protected. The states refer variously to "live premature child," "any unborn or aborted child," "embryo," "a human conceptus," and "the product of conception." Some states allow experimentation in order to diagnose a disease of the mother or to preserve the mother's or embryo's health. Most forbid the sale, transfer, or distribution of embryos or fetuses for improper uses; some forbid the sale of fetuses for experimentation.

In the pluralist American system, other policies at both the national and state levels provide a backdrop for monitoring IVF. Existing criminal, commercial, and civil codes can apply to embryo trafficking;[94] criminal codes can penalize fraud or dishonesty by IVF practitioners; and federal regulations on the use of human subjects in research can protect individuals used in experimental IVF protocols. Other executive agencies propose regulations to meet problems as they arise. The Food and Drug Administration, for example, recommended in February 1988 that fresh semen no longer be used in donor insemination because the AIDS virus could be transmitted to recipients. Instead, semen will be frozen and the donor will be tested for the AIDS virus six months later. Six months is thought to be the "window" for the virus of the time between exposure to the virus and its detection in tests. If the window is subsequently found to be longer, the FDA can easily extend the time of freezing.

Summary: Regulatory Policy. Regulatory policy ought to be enacted carefully, incrementally, and with a clear idea of the targeted benefits of regulation. Just as there should be agreed upon and stringent criteria for outright bans (e.g., an activity will be barred only if it poses a clear and present danger of intruding on a compelling state interest), so should there be agreed upon criteria for time, place, and manner restrictions. As the experiences in Massachusetts, Louisiana, and Illinois show, the intentions of lawmakers are not always met in the enactment of policies. At present and in the absence of crises, delayed policy is preferable to sporadic laws with ill-defined language that fail to meet their original purposes and may even have unintended and unwanted impacts.

In vitro fertilization is vulnerable as a sacrificial issue that absorbs the ire legislators feel toward abortion policies. One can conclude that IVF is presently defined in state legislatures and the U.S. Congress as an embryo's issue. While protecting the embryo is a legitimate state interest, protecting it above all other interests diverts attention in a nonconstructive way. Under Supreme Court decisions, fetuses do not have the rights of persons. It follows logically that embryos, which are considerably less developed than fetuses, also are without the constitutional rights of persons. Thus, to penalize IVF because it manipulates embryos might raise provocative moral questions but it is without legal grounding.

A preferred course of action is to shift attention from the embryo's rights to the clinical practice of IVF and to the interests of patients, who *are* persons under the law. If done incrementally, this will involve four steps. First, the private sector will assume the initiative in monitoring itself and developing minimal standards for the clinical practice of basic and expanded IVF. Self-monitoring will include (1) timely publication of guidelines, (2) specific steps to ensure high quality practice (e.g., minimal standards for membership in SART), (3) regular gathering and analyzing of data in order early to detect harms from basic and expanded IVF, and (4) prompt communication of harms and possible causes to physicians, patients, and the public. Self-monitoring will be conducted with central goals in mind, including the protection of patients from exploitative and dangerous practices and the protection of unborn children from unnecessary risks taken in order to expand services to couples.

Second, state health boards or legislatures will devise a method of periodically monitoring the effectiveness of voluntary regulation by the private sector. Ideally, this will be done with the cooperation of medical facilities. The state officials will determine if IVF clinics in that state report to the medical registry and adhere to recommendations made by professional groups in the private sector. They will also provide a forum in which former or potential IVF patients can air grievances related to their treatment at clinics in the state.

Third, where voluntary compliance is found to be ineffective, standards developed in the private sector can be codified in state law. This might include, for example, the licensing of laboratories that perform egg fertilizations and embryo freezing in the same way that states now license laboratories and personnel involved in performing semen or blood analysis.[95] The need for taking action will increase in states where practitioners do not comply with minimum standards recommended by medical groups. The first priority is to introduce quality control in the physical facilities. As a lawyer in Los Angeles put it, "Right now, there's nothing to prevent the deli across the street from sticking a liquid-nitrogen tank next to the pastrami and calling itself a sperm bank."[96] Similarly, no licensing regulations are now in effect regarding IVF and embryo cryopreservation laboratories. If the safety of patients and unborn children is a primary goal, this action is of top priority where practitioners are not following the counsel of their peers.

Fourth, the first states to license or otherwise regulate IVF facilities will then act as innovators in the state by state modeling that is a feature of American politics. At some point this modeling will be made formal in uniform state laws proposed by organizations that specialize in formulating codes for states to follow.

This clinically oriented, incremental approach uses the observations of IVF practitioners and patients to identify specific ways consumers can be hurt by today's practice of basic and expanded IVF. It puts the initiative in the private sector where, one assumes, exploitative or dangerous practices can be identified early and before harmful practices become routine. Placing the incentive to monitor in the hands of physicians arguably minimizes bureaucratic inertia. It was the private sector, for example, that developed the Registry for IVF data compiled by Medical Research International. The utility of the first MRI report, published in *Fertility and Sterility*,[97] is shown by the frequency with which the collected data have been cited in hearings and in other commentary. In contrast, no apparent benefit has come from IVF record-keeping required by law in Pennsylvania. No attempts have been made to analyze the data or to use them to monitor compliance with IVF standards of operation.[98] The workability of power-sharing between the medical community and policymakers is illustrated by the recent contract reached between the National Institutes of Health (NIH) and the MRI, in which the NIH supports continued data gathering by the MRI.[99]

An incremental model complements traditional methods of policymaking in this country. Incrementalism may have its drawbacks,[100] but, as an inherent part of the American policy context, it can be effectively used to oversee new reproductive technologies. At this point it is desirable to develop a feeling of competence in our ability to monitor and control these technologies. Incremental policy, starting in the private sector and spreading outward in state to state modeling to enhance quality control in IVF facilities, can create a record of small, concrete successes and reassert an expectation of the societal ability to manage rapidly changing technologies. It will help dethrone IVF from its current image as an unmanageable and untouchable political issue. It also creates time during which policymakers can narrow their focus to essential issues and search for authenticity in ways that will encourage useful long-term policy in the future. The plea to "do something" must be answered by a grounding in today's political and medical reality.

AFFIRMATIVE POLICY

Governments can also "do something" in the affirmative sense of promoting or aiding reproductive technologies. Affirmative policy eases techniques symbolically, by placing the weight of the government behind them, or pragmatically, by allocating resources for their use. The prospect of affirmative policy challenges society to set priorities, question values, and make decisions about its commitment to expanded IVF.

Affirmative policy presents the opportunity to ask whether approval, services and financial inducements ought to be given to laboratory conception. Unlike regulations, where crises often demand immediate answers, with affirmative policy, the luxury exists of reaching a consensus about the desirability of action before steps are actually taken. The questions for which consensus is sought are several. Should access to basic IVF for patients be facilitated? Should access to expanded IVF (egg and embryo freezing and donation) be facilitated? Should access to techniques designed to assure healthier children (for example, embryo biopsies) be facilitated when the techniques are available? If facilitation is desirable, what form should it take? Is it desirable to mandate insurance coverage of the techniques? Is it desirable to use public funds to cover the costs? In addition to asking whether patients should be helped to use laboratory conception, one can also ask about practitioners. Should they be helped, through federal grants, in their efforts to expand and improve IVF services?

Conferring Legitimacy. The government confers legitimacy on issues when it decides to regulate them. Turn-of-the-century child labor laws, for example, conferred legitimacy on the idea that the government would act as a substitute parent to protect children. A commission appointed after the Tuskegee syphilis study came to light, in which medical treatment had been deliberately withheld from men suffering from syphilis, conferred legitimacy on the issue of protecting human subjects of medical research.[101] In vitro fertilization, in contrast, has operated in the absence of this symbolic allocation of legitimacy. An important implication of the EAB's disbanding was the message that reproductive techniques had not achieved the status of a matter worthy of systematic discussion.

One affirmative policy, then, is to establish a national commission for the review and discussion of new reproductive technologies. Features of such a commission are discussed later in this chapter, so at this point the symbolic importance of a commission will simply be mentioned. Irrespective of what a national commission recommends, and whether it is basically sympathetic to new technologies or not, an important impact of a commission is to place the weight of the government behind the matter as one warranting discussion.

Other policies that would confer legitimacy on IVF fall under the general heading of "headache reduction." Here state or national policymakers would clarify ambiguities in the law that are disincentives for physicians and citizens who want to use the new technologies, such as silences about who is related to whom when donor tissues are used. They would also remove from the books or clarify the meanings of state fetal/embryo research laws that chill IVF practice or lead practitioners to believe they must practice IVF in certain restrictive ways, such as transferring all embryos even when doing so goes against medical judgment.

Clarification of these laws would ease access to IVF and indicate that policymakers are concerned about the impacts of vaguely written laws.

Financial Entitlement. Is it in society's best interest to make infertility and IVF treatment affordable to couples through the enactment of laws that mandate insurance coverage of treatments? After years in which couples have paid for IVF largely out of their own pockets, state governments have taken early steps to mandate insurance coverage. These laws call into question restrictive provisions such as this exclusion in a Health Maintenance Organization: "Infertility Services excluded are . . . invitro [sic] fertilization, embryo transplants, and other procedures deemed to be experimental or investigational in nature by any appropriate technological assessment body established by any state or federal government."

Infertile couples have taken the lead in changing insurance laws to prevent this type of exclusion. They were behind legislation in Maryland, which was the first state to revise insurance laws to recognize infertility as a medical condition and IVF as a treatment. Under the new Maryland law, married couples are entitled to some reimbursement for IVF if they have been infertile for five years or have infertility due to endometriosis, DES exposure, or blocked or missing fallopian tubes; tried less costly treatments unsuccessfully; used their own gametes; and tried IVF at centers conforming to AFS and ACOG standards.[102] The law does not extend to self-insured groups or to federal or city workers. Efforts to restrict coverage to 5 IVF cycles were unsuccessful; insurers falling under the scope of the law must offer benefits to the same extent as for treatments relating to pregnancy.[103]

Shortly after Maryland passed its law, Texas enacted a nearly identical law. Massachusetts followed with a broader law mandating insurance coverage for infertility treatment in general. In 1987 the Arkansas legislature enacted a law specifically including embryo freezing and setting a maximum benefit for IVF coverage at $15,000. Legislation passed in Hawaii in 1987 provides for a one-time-only IVF reimbursement.[104]

Incremental policy has taken hold with state-by-state modeling in the matter of financial entitlement. At the federal level, Representative Patricia Schroeder of Colorado introduced bills in the 100th Congress to provide benefits for federal employees and members of the uniformed services who adopt children and to provide benefits for federal employees who use "family-building procedures." Senator Alan Cranston of California introduced a bill to provide benefits to veterans with service-related infertility.[105] Ironically, considering that infertility treatment has during the 1980s centered mainly on women, infertility benefits for men have attracted Congressional attention. Cranston's bill was the only one of the above to make it out of committee in the 100th Congress, although it was dropped when Senate House conferees could not agree on language. Also, it was a letter from the chair of the Senate Committee on Veterans' Affairs that helped draw attention to the need for a study of Infertility Prevention and Treatment by the U.S. Congress Office of Technology Assessment.[106]

Health care coverage for IVF makes the technique accessible to different income groups and helps remedy today's situation in which only moderate and high income groups realistically can afford IVF, either because they have the money up front or have more comprehensive insurance coverage.[107] At one IVF center, 71 percent of the women and 80 percent of the men had more than a high school education, and most were dual income families.[108] Such signs of inequitable access to IVF have long caused concern for IVF supporters who believe that something more equitable than the action of the marketplace should dictate who has access to IVF. Insurance coverage also brings parity between medical care for fertility and infertility related conditions, as in Maryland's law, which requires insurers to grant IVF benefits "to the same extent as benefits provided for other pregnancy-related procedures."

There are, however, unanswered questions about affirmative policy. First, it is not clear what priority ought to be placed on infertility control as a societal goal. Daniel Callahan, an ethicist, holds the view that infertility ought to have low priority in our society. He writes: "Infertility is not a problem that cripples us as a society. We are not underpopulated. On the contrary, we already have too many children being born under less than desirable circumstances."[109] "It is not a proper goal of medicine," wrote Paul Ramsey, "to enable women to have children and marriages to be fertile *by any means.*"[110] How important a societal goal is it to help couples overcome infertility? It would be the single most important priority if 100 percent of our population were infertile. What, however, is the value when only 10 percent is infertile?[111] Where in our scheme of medical priorities does the treatment of infertility fit?

Second, even if one decides that infertility warrants attention, one must ask whether IVF coverage is the best way of committing resources. Perhaps it is preferable for the government to pursue the alternatives of encouraging and aiding adoptions, helping couples to see themselves and their lives as worthy even if childless, and allocating money and services to the prevention of infertility.[112] Although preventing infertility would require thoughtful and multifaceted policy, in the long run it might be more cost-efficient and less troublesome for couples than waiting for the infertility to manifest itself and then developing high technology solutions. The enthusiasm for IVF must not mask the knowledge that some cases of infertility are preventable in the first place.[113]

Third, there is an increasingly compelling voice in bioethics that challenges the wisdom of allocating resources to medical problems that are "unfortunate" but not "unfair."[114] A growing number of scholars question the use of sophisticated techniques when basic health needs languish and worsen. Early in IVF's history, Leon Kass criticized IVF as "yet another instance of our thoughtless preference for expensive high-technology, therapy-oriented approaches to disease and dysfunctions."[115] Putting the weight of the government behind insurance coverage for infertility will create feelings of entitlement to reproductive techniques at a time when, some authors believe, we should be dampening and not whetting the public appetite for a technological "fix."[116] Insurance coverage would also insulate patients and the public from the costs of techniques in a way that reduces public awareness of the consequences of the technologies they seek.[117]

Insurance coverage for basic IVF is a first step and demands for it can reasonably be expected to grow as the accordian of techniques unfolds in expanded IVF. It is important to think long and hard about the implications of extending entitlement to a vigorously growing new medical field. Insurance coverage must be crafted narrowly and with attention to the message of entitlement it conveys. Once again, there is a need for authenticity in the reasons for framing affirmative policy. Emotionalism has no more place in crafting affirmative policy than in regulatory policy, yet there are dangers that motherhood and babies will be used as provocative symbols for legislators. In the 1984 U.S. Congressional hearings, mothers of babies conceived during IVF stood for the legislators.[118] A lawyer involved in the Maryland insurance bill described the impact of the testimony of IVF patients during the committee hearings in that state:

"The dynamic was that they were asking the legislators if they could parent. The issue was motherhood. The high point came when the eighth or ninth woman spoke. She told the story of her infertility. And then she announced she was pregnant through the help of IVF. The committee applauded. There was not a dry eye in the audience. The impact was tremendous."

Fourth, mandated insurance coverage opens questions about reproductive rights that society may not yet be prepared to answer. By offering IVF to married couples using their own gametes and to couples with

104

demonstrated infertility, for example, Massachusetts and Texas simultaneously opened access and closed it. Widespread debate has not yet been generated about whether IVF should be available to single persons as well as to married persons or to fertile couples using donated tissues for genetic reasons as well as to infertile couples. Although virtually all laws "discriminate" by creating classifications, some create invidious discriminations that violate the 14th Amendment equal protection clause of the Constitution. Society must be prepared to grapple with the claims relating to reproductive rights. Should the right to conceive be given a liberal sweep to include single and married, gay and straight, fertile and infertile alike? Or should it be limited on the basis of marital status, purpose, and medical history? When insurance laws impose limitations, have invidious discriminations been created? Efforts to affirm IVF must be taken with ideas about the scope of the right to conceive in mind.

Fifth, automatic insurance coverage of IVF's variations shortens the "incubation" period during which the variation is monitored for safety and effectiveness. Arkansas, for example, sets a lifetime maximum infertility coverage at $15,000. This presumably can be spent in any way the couple sees fit, which would include tissue donations or freezing. Arguably, however, this quick integration of tissue freezing into the umbrella of insured IVF procedures sidesteps an opportunity to examine freezing's benefits, prematurely removes the burden of demonstrating safety from the medical community, and gives the message to patients that freezing is accepted and beneficial. When IVF variations are accepted as reimbursable, a pattern is set in which the goodness of the techniques is accepted without an open, public review of their clinical practice.

Federal Funding. Researchers and clinicians make a persuasive claim for federal funding of IVF research. A survey of IVF directors showed that the vast majority favored it.[119] The British and Australian governments review and fund research involving human embryos. In the United States, the disbanding of the EAB has created a de facto moratorium on federal funding. An affirmative policy would end this moratorium, either by changing the policy of the Department of Health and Human Services so that IVF research no longer needs EAB approval, reinstating the EAB, or starting fresh with a new review board.[120]

Research on the conditions of IVF will occur with or without the federal funding of projects. The tug of professional curiosity and the desire to understand and improve IVF lead researchers to study IVF with funds generated by patient fees, donations by patients, hospital operating funds, and grants by pharmaceutical and other companies. At present, research using human embryos takes several forms. One is the correlational study, in which technicians observe and statistically analyze the conditions under which fertilization, cleavage, and implantation take place. The embryo itself is not manipulated. Results are communicated in the professional literature and through workshops in order to maximize IVF's effectiveness.

In other studies technicians study eggs that do not fertilize or that fertilize and are nonviable. The tissues would not be transferred to the woman in any event and they do not have the potential of becoming human. Manipulations on these tissues are not thought to present a moral problem. An example is the study (and destruction) of polyspermic eggs; i.e., eggs fertilized by more than one spermatozoan, which makes them abnormal.[121] In other, much rarer, studies technicians manipulate (and destroy) normal embryos that could become human. These embryos are either left over from IVF and donated by patients or are created from donor eggs and sperm for the purpose of research. An example is to study these embryos for chromosomal abnormalities in order to investigate the safety of IVF.[122] The prospect of creating embryos for research purposes has raised concern among observers. Of eleven commissions making recommendations about the matter from around the world, ten accepted the principle of studying embryos left over and donated during IVF, but only four accepted the principle of creating embryos for study.[123]

Funding research for any of these types of studies would have the advantage of helping to remedy today's ironic situation in which research is, in effect, conducted on patients as they go through IVF rather than in controlled studies before clinical interaction.[124] This pattern was set in the years following Pierre Soupart's proposal. He had wanted to obtain eggs from women undergoing sterilization, fertilize them, and examine them for chromosomal abnormalities. In the aftermath of the EAB report, neither his study nor any other was conducted. Instead, on the basis of successful births, practitioners started offering IVF and refining it as they went along.

A similar situation occurred in Australia, where one practitioner proposed to test the safety of freezing eggs, which is more difficult than freezing embryos because eggs are less developed and more delicate. To test the safety of egg freezing, eggs need to be frozen, thawed, fertilized, examined for abnormalities, and discarded. The Standing Review and Advisory Committee, a board set up by law in the state of Victoria to review projects using human embryos, turned down the proposal.[125] Despite the lack of published studies attesting to the safety of egg freezing in humans, clinicians have begun egg freezing. In Australia and Germany infants have been born from embryos made up of frozen and thawed eggs.[126]

One of two things can happen when preparatory research using human tissues is not considered for funding. The practice to be studied (e.g., egg freezing) can be put on hold until public attitudes change, or the practice can be refined in the clinical setting with patients as subjects. That the second has happened says something about the physician's push to study and the patient's yearning to consume. A danger is that even if the government does begin to fund embryo research projects, the pattern of innovating without rigorous pretesting by researchers in independent settings will become difficult to unseat.

If the government were to review grant proposals in IVF, it would invite a new level of scrutiny of researchers who presently need to receive only permission of review boards within their home institutions. In some cases in-house review is cursory. If the review committee decides a practice is a clinical application and not research, as in the start of embryo freezing programs, review may not even be required. Even if the practice is reviewed, in-house peers, as colleagues of the researchers, are not necessarily the most critical of reviewers.[127] Further, researchers in private, nonuniversity settings are not even obligated to have this kind of peer review.

With government funding, proposals would pass internal review and then be scrutinized in a second review by scientists within the granting agencies. This opens proposals to a level of the independent review by specialized experts. Where a proposal is turned down, the applicants are effectively informed that features of their proposed method or purpose need rethinking and improvement. This additional review makes federal funding a double-edged sword for the researcher. It brings in dollars to support research but also opens the project to regulation and control.[128] As a result, not all IVF practitioners favor federal involvement. Instead some prefer the status quo, fearing that "He who pays the piper calls the tune," and "with money comes power."

Proponents of federal funding argue that it will advance knowledge by lifting the cloud now cast upon research using human embryos. Among other things supporters predict that tomorrow's research will advance the understanding of and solutions to embryo loss in IVF, male infertility, miscarriages, contraception, and genetic defects in embryos.[129] Opinion polls show support for research dealing with such topics. An opinion poll conducted in late 1986 revealed a large percentage of the public sampled

(82 percent) supported research in biotechnology and genetic engineering.[130] Eighty-three percent supported gene manipulations to correct genetic diseases.

Opening IVF research would also help prevent what appears to be an emerging inauthenticity. When asked about the prospects for human embryo research in this country, IVF practitioners are chary about the topic: "It is a sticky issue," "I don't see embryo research ever taking place in the United States, at least not as public knowledge," "No one will do it; the press pressure would close down the clinics." Yet researchers are studying embryos. Freezing programs put options in their consent forms for couples to donate their embryos for research, nonviable embryos are studied, and ad hoc research is ongoing that will produce information useful for IVF. Researchers in Europe have studied viable embryos, created embryos for the sole purpose of research, and published the results of their findings.[131] That practitioners are so skittish about talking about who in this country might be conducting research using human embryos indicates that the topic is slipping to the realm of secrecy and dissembling, neither of which is helpful in an area already hulking under secrecy and defensiveness.

It would not be an unmitigated blessing for the government to open its doors to IVF and embryo research, however. For one thing, it will open the door to linear consumption of new techniques which, as this book argues, is not necessarily a societal good. One senses from reading about visions for what can be done if embryo research were politically acceptable that the stage is being set for a rapid unfolding of scientific inquiry once governmental approval is given. The literature contains the metaphor of IVF and embryo study as the steps "up" to a field of positive consequences. The metaphor is rich with movement: IVF is thought to be a "window" to greater knowledge and the embryo is the "vehicle" for that ascent.[132] The acceleration takes a 'jump and soar" character in which the study of embryos will open the window for the resolution of infertility (jump) and much, more more (soar). With IVF, for example:

In vitro fertilization . . . has provided opportunities which if developed with understanding and skill will provide great benefits for society in general.[133]

The potential benefits of IVF extend far beyond the relief of infertility.[134]

There are undoubtedly other as yet unimagined areas in which research on human pre-embryos will offer clinical advantages.[135]

The same kind of demand creation that took place with basic infertility, where the public rather suddenly started hearing of an infertility epidemic, desperate women, and ticking biological clocks, is echoed in the literature on embryo research. There are said to be "pressing reasons"[136] and an "urgent need" to proceed with research that will at some point require the study of human embryos. Studies of human embryos provide the "essential bridge" between research using animals and clinical applications with humans. If embryo research is not conducted, society must bear a "price-tag" in the form of "lost" or "foregone" knowledge.[137] The knowledge will benefit growing numbers of people in accelerating ways. The "unborn patient" will benefit if genetic defects can be detected in the embryonic state.[138] In the more distant future, persons with cancer, diabetes, and other diseases will reap the rewards of knowledge gained by the study of embryos. Gene therapy, which will allow modification of genetic defects in embryos, will reduce human suffering.[139] In short, to open embryo research for federal funding is to unleash a spectrum of tantalizing visions.

Another problem with funding for embryo research is its impact on societal sensibilities. Current restrictions against embryo research are justified on the grounds that the human embryo is a powerful symbol in our society that needs protection.[140] If one adheres to the idea that the embryo as symbol should be protected, one would find embryo research unsettling. Researchers who systematically study embryos categorize and judge them, either using "reject" embryos from IVF, or creating embryos for study from donated eggs and sperm. When it becomes politically acceptable to conduct embryo research, researchers will need to create them in large numbers in order to assure scientifically valid results.

The creation, grading, and discarding of embryos is, when compared with child abuse, murders, war, and other casualties of modern life, arguably a minor matter. The embryos are, after all, microscopic, fragile, merely potential human life, and are lost by the millions in the natural order of things where embryos pass from women's bodies with no sign they ever existed. Still, one could argue that deliberate experimentation is yet another thing to assault the sensibilities of a society jaded by the dual attraction and repulsion of xenografts (transfer of animal organs to humans), "farming" of recently deceased anencephalic infants for organs, five-organ transplants, and fetal tissue transplants for diseased patients. Embryo research is, seen in this light, just one more step toward the suspicion that very little is sacrosanct in modern-day medicine. In short, an alternative to funding of embryo research is for researchers and scientists not to reach for the carrot and to pause in their consumption until it is clearly decided that the need is "pressing" and "urgent."

Summary: Affirmative Policy. Affirmative policy is at a juncture, which gives interested citizens the chance to make deliberate decisions about whether and how society should allocate symbolic and financial resources for expanded IVF. Insurance coverage, headache reduction laws, and research funding would send a message of legitimacy about IVF and the choices of expanded IVF. This would encourage consumption and entitlement claims. The escalator up is as compelling a metaphor in the 1990s as was the slippery slope down in the 1970s. Before building affirmative policy, we need to examine the stated benefits just as carefully as we examine the stated dangers before moving ahead with regulatory policy.

Toward this end, agreed upon criteria are needed to evaluate the anticipated benefit. Here the clear and present danger standard for regulatory policy can be used as a model. Before funding research or extending health care benefits, it makes sense to look at the degree and likelihood of benefit. Who will benefit from this proposed policy? What is the likelihood of benefit? When will the benefit be felt? Is the benefit an end in itself or a means to a benefit further in the future? It is desirable to develop a formulation that says a proposed application is acceptable only if there is a clear, present, and self-contained benefit to a specific group of individuals with a compelling need.

An incremental approach to affirmative policy can be pursued in which benefits are sought in a small, concrete, and bounded manner. The impact of this policy will be examined and, if it is appropriate, will be expanded in the same kind of modeling as for regulatory policy. Research funding might be appropriate, for example, only for projects designed clearly to relieve a specific clinical burden on patients; i.e., a study to test different media for the incubation of embryos during IVF. Or reimbursement in insurance coverage might be appropriate only for couples with demonstrated infertility, for a set number of attempts, to a dollar maximum, and for attempts at centers meeting rigorous standards of quality control.

The task is to be wary about "created" and tantalizing demands. We must ask: is the benefit clear and present or merely vague and futuristic? Along what path does the escalator up direct us? To resolving cancer? Preventing birth defects? Improving fertility treatment? The stated benefits travel along different avenues. Which of the many avenues do we want to pursue? How will we set priorities? Why do we resist advancing one step at a time?

INACTION

I naction or policy deferral suggests either that the government is too caught up in the politics of the matter to act or that a choice has been made to leave matters to existing policy and medical self-regulation. As argued throughout this chapter, inaction for reasons of political stalemate is not valid. Inaction as a deliberate form of benign neglect, however, is appropriate inasmuch as it reflects a policy choice. When one compares the context of constitutional protection for procreational freedoms sanctioned by the Supreme Court with hostility of the legislature to IVF, one can conclude that inaction has to this point not necessarily harmed reproductive technologies. The Supreme Court's decisions acknowledging constitutionally based rights not to conceive and not to bear children suggest broad ranging rights on matters relating to childbearing. Without a specific decision to the contrary, it is generally presumed that the right *not* to procreate subsumes a right *to* procreate.[141]

The Supreme Court has built a congenial constitutional backdrop on matters of procreation. Over the years, the Court has affirmed a broad individual liberty in raising children, having children, not conceiving children, and not bearing children.[142] It has called procreation "one of the basic civil rights of man" and a "basic liberty."[143] In a decision dealing with access to contraceptives, the Court stated:

If the right of privacy means anything, it is the right of the individual, married or single, to be free from unwarranted government intrusion into matters so fundamentally affecting a person as the decision whether to bear or beget a child.[144]

In the first of several opinions establishing a woman's right to end her pregnancy, the Court stated that the right of privacy, grounded in 14th Amendment liberty, was "broad enough to encompass a woman's decision whether or not to terminate her pregnancy."[145] This principle has withstood continued assaults by state legislatures and city governments. Still, the steady challenges to the abortion decisions, statements by individual Justices, nuances of recent Court decisions, and efforts by the Reagan administration to limit access of young people to contraceptives suggest that the field is becoming or will become less congenial to the expansion of procreational liberties. If this is the case, the argument for letting matters stand takes on even greater potency.

THE RESPONSIBLE GOVERNMENT

The history of governmental involvement has been one of inauthenticity characterized by a tendency to hide from conflict and to focus on fetuses, embryos, Xeroxed humans—everything but the issue at hand, which is whether the public sector ought to assert control over the practice of basic and expanded IVF and whether public resources ought to be used to ease access to IVF. The responsible government will attempt to achieve authenticity. This means, most importantly, establishing a forum for open and frank discussions of the conflicting societal values about new conceptions.

A Forum for Discussion. In the 1984 hearings on embryo transfer in the U.S. Congress, witnesses spoke with "remarkable unanimity"[146] of the need to set up a national body to review, oversee, and educate citizens about new reproductive technologies. One can feel sympathy for the reaction, "What, another commission?" to this suggestion. Criticisms are leveled against national commissions as being excuses for more talk and less action. National commissions are variously said to be ways of "smothering problems," "part of government by fire brigade," and the stage for "a kind of Alice in Wonderland—with the same moving picture re-shown over and over again, the same analysis, the same recommendations, and the same inaction."[147] Because commission members from varied disciplines are called upon to reach a consensus about controversial matters, commission reports can end up as case studies in "studious avoidance," reflecting little analytic rigor.[148]

On the other hand, commissions have effectively mobilized attention and directed debate in the past.[149] A commission can be a useful starting point for societal discussion about a controversial matter. As to the criticism that it means more talk and less action, delayed policy is preferable to premature and hastily conceived policy. One wonders if action without talk has anything to be said in its favor in any event.

As with consumption of IVF and research in general, one can also ask in the public context about policy, "what's the rush?" A strong case can be made for a slow, thoughtful evolution of policy (what is commonly called "muddling through" or "incrementalism"), especially in an area with as strong an emotional legacy as IVF. Incrementalism is described by Charles Lindblom, a political scientist, as follows: "It is decision-making through small or incremental moves on particular problems rather than through a comprehensive reform program. It is also endless; it takes the form of an infinite sequence of policy moves. Moreover, it is exploratory in that the goals of policy-making continue to change as new experience with policy throws new light on what is possible and desirable."[150]

In a different context, Harry Krause, a law professor, calls for a similar kind of incremental "building-up" in the area of IVF: "I suggest we work "inductively" from concrete cases up, rather than "deductively" from abstract principles down. I suggest that, in the common law tradition, we deal intelligently with concrete, *micro* problems and let the *macro* picture develop from there."[151]

Incrementalism as a model, however, ought not to be allowed to develop helter-skelter. As Abram and Wolf put it, "Ad hoc decisions all over the map, in a world without substantive or procedural regularity, will guarantee error and conflict."[152] The role of a national commission is to provide a direction for that incrementalism. A commission (most recommendations are that it be temporary, removed from political appointments, neutral, interdisciplinary, and advisory only) would bring together resources, educate the government, generate public debate, and provide a forum for common standards and areas of accord.[153] It would help as we as a society try to "articulate the moral ground we share and to try to enlarge it."[154] An alternative to the commission is the consensus conference, a meeting conducted by a federal agency such as the National Institutes of Health, in which experts reach a consensus regarding the scientific efficacy and safety of IVF and related techniques.[155]

The argument in this chapter is that policy ought to be built gradually and carefully from voluntary regulation, state by state modeling, and, if needed, federal legislation. Throughout, however, the federal government must take the initiative in creating one or more forums for public discussion about IVF. A responsible government will provide guidance in its roles as mediator and forum-provider.

Guidance for Discussion. The discussion ideally will help governors and governed see IVF as an issue with its own merits. This means separating it from the barnacle issues of abortion, Nazism, and cloning, all of which are highly emotional and divert attention from the specific issues of IVF, which are worthy in their own right, such as honesty in the clinical practice of IVF, allocation of insurance resources to IVF treatment, and the question of whether new family relations ought to be clarified in state law.

It is also important to demystify IVF and defuse some of the red flags surrounding it. In vitro fertilization is not a miracle cure nor an instrument for producing monster babies; it is instead a clinical interaction between doctor and patient, albeit one that raises societal implications. Certainly some emotionalism generates interest in the subject and is a valuable indicator of the strength of public opinion. Too much emotionalism simply detracts, however. The government must not substitute new volatile symbols (e.g., sanctification of motherhood in hearings on insurance) for old red flags (e.g., test-tube babies, photocopied humans).

The discussion should be aimed at resolving the priorities about infertility as a medical issue before moving on to expanded IVF. It is important that IVF and infertility not be shuffled to the background before we understand our attitudes about them. Quite possibly reproductive technologies will mobilize more public support once people realize tissue freezing and examination of embryos for chromosomal defects will increase the options of fertile couples in making life-style choices and preventing birth defects. Political realism dictates that infertility, with its relatively small numbers of silent, female constituents, is not a top priority in state and federal legislatures. Realism also suggest that expanded IVF, with its prospects for a larger and more active constituency, will gradually become a higher priority.

It is important to develop an appropriate model for sharing authority between the private and public sectors. Toward this end, the debate should be geared to weighing several questions. First, should the effort to conceive be regarded primarily as a private matter or a public matter? If a private matter, governmental regulation should be minimal in order to avoid intrusion into a couple's personal decisions about when and how to have children. This places authority in the medical community for monitoring itself and suggests that attention should be given to improving the nature of the physician/patient interchange in order to reform the practice of IVF. If alternative conception is seen as a public matter, on the other hand, governmental oversight is encouraged in order to protect societal interests threatened by new conceptions.

Related to this is the question of how efforts to conceive fit into the society's tradition of reproductive freedom. If the Supreme Court has recognized as part of constitutional privacy and liberty a couple's decision *not* to conceive or bear children, does this mean the couple's decision *to* conceive is accorded equal constitutional protection? Are the rights not to conceive and to conceive, in other words, equally reverse sides of procreational freedom? If so, efforts to regulate IVF that reduce a couple's access to it must be done only for compelling reasons and the government's role should be minimal. If the right to conceive is seen as substantively different (among other things, it involves people other than the couple and it includes the interests of unborn children), a justification less stringent than "compelling" might suffice for regulatory policy to be enacted. Here the government's authority is greater.

Third, what is a desirable timetable for policy? A strong case can be made for waiting until more of the new conceptions are developed and practiced. Delayed policy will help prevent "instant obsolescence," in which policy is outdated soon after framing.[156] It will also give IVF time to mature as an issue. The current pluralistic blend of attentive groups is not necessarily an accurate reflection of social interests. The most active groups are the right to life groups and medical organizations, with patient consumer groups only recently beginning to take hold. This means a relatively passive majority supports new conceptions and a vocal minority opposes them. With time, a greater interplay of social groups seems likely.

Delaying policy has the disadvantage, however, of leaving consumers unprotected. If, for example, the states eventually license egg fertilization and embryo freezing laboratories, consumers using facilities with suboptimal conditions will be injured in the meantime by what might turn out to have been been preventably low success rates. In addition, undesirable patterns of interaction between physician and patient might become entrenched and difficult to dislodge if reforms are delayed. The question, in short, is when the mantle should be passed from private to public oversight. Should the medical community be in charge until more types of new conceptions unfold? Or should policymakers enter early in the evolution of the techniques?

Fourth, should IVF be approached with a strategy of short-term, ad hoc, and incremental policy? Or should an effort at long-term planning be undertaken? Is it better to take action now and build slowly from it, as in taking a grain of sand (a small policy innovation) and building a "pearl" of policy, layer by layer from it? Or is it better to make reasonable projections about future techniques and develop comprehensive policy with predicted implications in mind? With the former might we lose sight of goals and societal implications?

Fifth, the debate needs to weigh the extent to which public distrust of the medical community colors attitudes about policy. Do we as a society believe in the slippery slope of horrendous applications at the hands of white-coated scientists? Do hidden beliefs about scientists affect public judgment about who is best qualified to oversee the new conceptions? In regard to public ambivalence toward technology,[157] do we draw the line on the side of trust or distrust? Is medical policymaking a desired alternative in a technological era?

The irony about setting a forum for public debate is that IVF for women seems to be for policymakers a dreary issue. One predicts that officials will become increasingly attentive as laboratory conception reaches more constituents and promises more benefits (e.g., preventing genetic defects that are costly to cure). Here laboratory conception takes on a new meaning—not a luxury to circumvent infertility but a preventive device to ward off diseases and defects. This may move policy ahead but it should not be done with one entire dimension of IVF left unanswered; namely, the question of whether the government should put its weight with either regulatory or affirmative policy behind conception for women with blocked fallopian tubes.

In summary, a responsible government will encourage discussion, data gathering, and policy forums with special attention to reaching a consensus about private/public power sharing, the timing of policy, the nature of the right to conceive, and attitudes about basic and expanded IVF. The potential for developing appropriate policy models is real only when the issue is taken seriously enough to take steps to build those models.

CHAPTER SIX

A Responsible Public

WITNESSING EXPANDED IVF

The world of reproductive technologies brings into society a smorgasbord laden with tempting dishes in which couples, doctors, scientists, and a fascinated public are the neophyte diners wondering which dish to try and when. This hardly meets the Brave New World image of test-tube babies and a palpable loss of freedom. In George Orwell's *1984*, party members bore children only through an artificial insemination ("artsem") program mandated and controlled by the government. Only the proletariat ("proles") could try sexual intercourse; party members Julia and Winston met their doom because of illicit trysts above the junk store.

In the actual year of 1984 procreational choice took several leaps when, in that single year alone, three events occurred. First, an infant was born in Australia that had been frozen as an embryo, thereby demonstrating that a human embryo could be frozen in a special cryoprotectant, thawed, and transferred without adverse effects.[1] Next, a baby was born through IVF with an egg donated from another woman, making it the first infant to have both a genetic mother (the egg donor) and gestational mother (the one who bore the child).[2] Then a baby was born that had been flushed, as an embryo, from the uterus of one woman and transferred to the uterus of another (ovum transfer), making it the first baby to have a genetic and gestational mother AND to have existed in the wombs of two different women.[3]

In 1986 a woman wrote to advice columnist Abigail van Buren:

Dear Abby: I am a post-menopausal woman who wants very much to have a baby with family genes. I am thinking about asking my unmarried 20-year-old daughter to have an egg fertilized ex utero by the sperm of my 18-year-old son.
Would this be incestuous?

Wondering[4]

"Wondering" (her signature was revealing) symbolizes the gradual dawning taking place among a small but growing number of citizens that new conceptions offer choice. In vitro fertilization is not just a technique performed on infertile women; its variations can and will be used by many people for reasons other than overcoming infertility. It provides a way of bypassing genetic defects or, as in the case of "Wondering," to stave off the effects of aging. When "Wondering" wrote her letter, a forty-eight-year old woman in South Africa was on the brink of becoming pregnant with triplets created through IVF with the eggs of her daughter and the sperm of her son-in-law.[5] Had the case of the world's first mother/grandmother occurred ten years before, the press and public would have been shocked and scandalized. Occurring in 1987, however, a kind of normalcy has set in in which the event does not jar or rattle, if one could take muted press coverage as a sign of aplomb. A routineness has set in whereby the reaction is more "what's next?" than an analysis of the event itself. Laboratory conception has become a fact that, even in its strangest variation, is less controversial than when Louise Brown was born in 1978.

New conceptions involve choices that both beckon and unsettle. Ironically, the one conception that has aroused public emotional involvement more than any other is a low-technology application—surrogate motherhood—in which women bear babies for contracting couples. Surrogacy in itself provokes public feelings and when something goes wrong with the arrangement, the intensity of involvement grows. In the case of *In re Baby M*, for example,[6] a surrogate, Mary Beth Whitehead, refused to give up the baby she had borne under contract for Elizabeth and William Stern. When the Sterns let her keep the baby for several days, she fled with the infant to another state. She was eventually brought back under court order. After the case went to court, a judge ordered custody for the Sterns with visitation rights for Whitehead. At one point before the hearing, Mr. Stern had taped a conversation with Whitehead, who asked "[S]o what do we do? Cut her in half?"[7] The infant, known as Melissa by the Sterns, Sara by the Whiteheads, and Baby M in the court and press, had been divided no less than had a confused public.

The public's trouble in fathoming surrogacy created divisive opinions, united only in the wish that this seemingly no-win situation had not come to be. In one cartoon, that penguin Opus, who lives in Bloom County, is suffering from a crisis of faith. Buffeted by revelations about illicit arms sales to Iran, Wall Street scandals, and sexual activities of evangelists, he asks the reader, "What can a fellow believe in anymore? Are there no more bastions of purity?" Spotting a pregnant woman, he rushes over and rests his cheek on her protruding stomach. He has found his answer. "Motherhood!" But the woman delivers the final blow. "Surrogate."[8]

Like abortion before it, surrogate motherhood swept IVF on its coat-tails. Surrogacy, when combined with egg, sperm, and embryo transfer, creates streams of parenthood possibilities in which a child can end up with as many as five "parents": a genetic mother, genetic father, gestational mother, social mother, and social father. Writers make charts outlining the combinations of the new conceptions.[9] One cartoonist shows a teacher writing a mathematical formulation on the board:

Donor   +
Surrogate mother   +
Contract   =
Exhibit A (baby)   ÷
Lawsuit   +
Media   +

A diminutive child watches in dismay. "Cripes! All I asked was 'Where did I come from?!' "[10] In another cartoon two children play in a sandbox. One explains to the other, "My mother was a surrogate who had in vitro fertilization from an unknown donor sanctioned by my Dad. How about you?" The other frets. "I don't know if I can handle the laughter when I tell him the stork brought me!"[11]

Through publicity, matters like the Baby M case that "touch" citizens' emotions, together with the sheer range of possibilities, signal that conception choices reach beyond infertile couples. Even the infertile as a constituency is growing as a result of the reduced social onus of infertility and the rise in physically based infertility. Among the potential users of tissue donation, freezing, or surrogate motherhood are persons who: (1) have jobs potentially dangerous for unborn children, (2) are about to undergo radiation or other medical therapy, (3) marry young and want to store gametes for later conception; (4) have a genetically related defect such as sickle-cell anemia, (5) want to store gametes before having a tubal ligation or vasectomy for birth control, and (6) are single and need egg, embryo, sperm, or uterus donors to conceive.

Thus, at least three "attentive publics" or constituencies either have wondered or will begin to wonder about choices available to them: infertile couples, persons who work in dangerous occupations or who fear their children will inherit genetic defects, and persons interested in exercising life-style choices such as postponed childbearing. Each may have reasons to use IVF, tissue donation, or genetic testing of embryos. Each has friends and family, who, by their vicarious interest, become part of the expanding attentive public. These constituencies differ from the public that watched over Louise Brown's birth as spectators transfixed by a new, distant, "gee-whiz" technique. These publics are attentive for personal reasons. Expanded IVF now touches people who want to exercise choice and who are potential participants.

DEVELOPING AN ETHIC OF CHOICE

As more citizens are touched by the field of reproductive technologies, they become involved in ethical thinking. Ethics, the study of the "rightness or wrongness of human conduct,"[12] involves choices. It deals with "public values" that "govern what one does or does not do when others are watching." Morals, in contrast, are internalized notions of right and wrong; they "govern what one does or does not do when no one is watching."[13] Ethics gives a handle for evaluating reproductive techniques and the role citizens play as potential consumers. Abigail van Buren told "Wondering" that her scheme "would be not only incestuous, it would be illegal, immoral and outrageous," but society would be hard pressed to rely on an advice columnist for standards of propriety.

The reproductive choices infiltrating society are like finger lakes wending their way into different corridors of the public. At first the lakes reached infertile couples; with expanded IVF they will reach couples in whose heritage lie genetic defects and tomorrow's adults who will want to exercise choice in their childbearing years. Even though the techniques are novel, the issues they raise are timeless: the nature of the family, the meaning of parenthood, the place of children in a society, and the balance of individual desires against social needs.[14]

As techniques have unfolded to this point, the government has avoided the issues, clinicians use their own models with medical criteria, and patients are preoccupied with their own struggle to conceive. Amid the inner-directedness of the participants, persons trained in biomedical ethics, philosophy, and theology have taken upon themselves the role of identifying criteria for evaluating basic and expanded IVF. Ethicists sit on government commissions, medical interest group committees, and specially constituted hospital ethics committees. The Department of Health, Education, and Welfare, for example, set up the *Ethics* Advisory Board; the American Fertility's Society's *Ethics* Committee produced the *"Ethical* Statement on In Vitro Fertilization" in 1984 and the *"Ethical* Considerations of the New Reproductive Technologies" in 1986; and the *Ethics* Committee of the American College of Obstetricians and Gynecologists produced the *"Ethical* Issues in Human In Vitro Fertilization and Embryo Placement" in 1986.

One turns to ethics to question the goodness of medical techniques and their method of administration. Should diners at the smorgasbord use cost/benefit principles of evaluation in deciding whether to return to the heating table (e.g., weighing the costs of indigestion against the benefits of satiation)? Or should they look to unchanging and universal moral principles (e.g., that glutttony is inherently a vice)? One also turns to ethics for a softening of the edges of medical technology. Ethics looks to the humanist values in medicine, which respect human dignity and evince concern for the "preservation, enhancement, fulfillment, and enrichment of human life." [15]

The ethicist (or philosopher or theologian) who ponders choice is like a sculptor walking round and round a clay statue in the making, examining its curves at leisure and trying to reach standards for gauging the wisdom of adding more clay here and chiseling more clay there. In IVF's early years, sensational headlines and superficial press coverage kept citizens at a distance from the statues and it relegated them to the status of persons on whirlwind tours of art museums who were able to judge each piece only with the help of captions and titles: "Babies Storm Growing," "Doctors Start Baby Outside the Womb." [16]

Ethics has invited more substantive self-awareness of the principles by which persons make choices about medical techniques. It also encourages a concern for the implications of those technologies on human dignity. Thus, all persons who focus on principles of choice become part of an ethical interchange. Individual decisions and choices, when taken as a whole, build a group and then societal ethic. To what, though, should we as citizens look in making choices? How can we become circumspect and principled consumers or, if not active participants, how can we help create an ambiance valuing limits on choice?

Moral Reasoning. In handling choice, should we as a public look for unyielding moral truths in the style championed by the late theologian Paul Ramsey? To Ramsey, "We must seek our rendezvous with some Nevers, and the good reasons for them."[17] One "Never" for Ramsey was experimentation on future human beings (embryos in IVF) which was, he reasoned, by the nature of things, immoral and illicit:

I must judge that in vitro fertilization constitutes unethical medical experimentation on possible future human beings, and therefore it is subject to absolute moral prohibition. I ask that my exact language be noted: I said, unethical experimentation on *possible future human beings.* By this, I mean the child-to-be, the "successful" experiments when they come.[18]

Recourse to moral thinking means using reason and analysis to uncover the inherent "rightness" of an act.[19] Here we must seek to make "correct moral decisions" about using new conceptions:[20]

Anticipation of possible legal and financial problems with in vitro fertilization can never absolve us from the responsibility of deciding whether this procedure is intrinsically right or wrong morally.[21]

Among the "self-evident truths" expressed is Ramsey's belief that experimentation on future human beings is immoral; the belief expressed by Pope Pius XII in 1956 that procreation, under natural law, must be based on a physical coupling between woman and man; and the conviction that creating hybrids between animals and humans would violate the natural order of things.[22] Analytically reached truths make their way into our history in, for example, the Declaration of Independence ("We hold these truths to be self-evident") and in Supreme Court decisions in which acts are proscribed if they offend common standards of decency or contradict Western sensibilities.[23]

Religious doctrine is another place to look for guidance about the inherent rightness of an act. The position of the Vatican, for example, is that the embryo is a person from the moment of conception and that this certainty precludes in vitro fertilization:

The human being is to be respected and treated as a person from the moment of conception; and therefore from that same moment his rights as a person must be recognized, among which in the first place is the inviolable right of every innocent human being to life.[24]

The inherent rightness or wrongness of new conceptions varies by religion and interpretation. Some theologians read certain biblical passages to mean that conception is a mysterious process decided by God and should not be tampered with by humans:

[T]hou it was who knitted me together in my mother's womb.—Psalms 139.13

You do not know how a pregnant woman comes to have a body and a living spirit in her womb; nor do you know how God the maker of things works.—Ecclesiastes[25]

Others, however, believe that the Bible contains a "profound endorsement for the vocation of parenthood, and an understanding of the human desire to become parents."[26] Among the passages they cite is this:

> Behold, sons are a gift from the Lord;
>   the fruit of the womb is a reward.
> Like arrows in the hand of a warrior are
>   the sons of one's youth.
> Happy the man whose quiver is filled with
>   them.—Psalms 127. 3–5.[27]

On the one hand, religion guides the making of decisions and it suggests the importance of looking to systematic principles for choice. It encourages people to consult criteria other than everyday need or wish. On the other hand, there is little evidence that it is a potent guide to action; persons trying IVF indicate little regard for religious teachings or they find a priest or minister willing to interpret religious doctrine in a way that permits new conceptions.

An alternative to using theological criteria for guiding choice is to use ad hoc intuition as a guide. This involves filtering out things that are unacceptable to the individual, to the community, and to society if there are shared values across different communities. Intuitive reactions invite emotions and "strong sentiments"[28] into decision making and they encourage observation of vaguely felt notions about what seems right and what does not. As the authors of the Warnock report put it, the ultimate question must be: "In what sort of society can we live with our conscience clear?"[29] An early example of intuitionism is described by Robert Edwards, who had a conversation with his department chair about his research on external human fertilization:

"It is unethical," she said.
"Why?" I asked.
"Because it is," she replied.[30]

Similarly, one writer condemned research on human embryos, saying the idea "leaves a nasty taste in the mouth."[31]

The problem with ad hoc intuition is that each person has idiosyncratic preferences; thus, there are as many intuitions as persons. Moreover, intuition invites the kinds of emotional reactions that have proved counterproductive in the debate over IVF. On the other hand, a certain degree of emotion helps invigorate the debate and keep it from becoming a recitation of scientific fact. Also, from these intuitions the earliest value building occurs and from them one can seek common standards of what, to a community of reasonable persons, will *not* do. With surrogacy, for example, a consensus is arising across societal groups that paying a woman to bear a child, with its implications of baby selling, "will *not* do." Intuition can also be used by individuals to make decisions about their own place in the consumption of new technologies.

Cost/Benefit Evaluation. Another way of evaluating new conceptions is to use cost/benefit reasoning to outline projected injuries and benefits of techniques. In contrast to the search for the Nevers, cost/benefit reasoning involves constant weighing of values; its outcome depends upon the particular situation and the values of that period of history. The scale is relative, not absolute, and the outcome is contingent on the context in which the balancing takes place.

As a rational method of inquiry, cost/benefit thinking meshes well with common methods in our society for reaching decisions based on empiricism, inference, and quantitatively based balance sheets. In its narrow form it is even codified in law in the form of mandated planning, programming, and budgeting analysis. In the field of IVF it would mean collecting data about risks to patients, embryos, and resulting children and weighing the desirability of that risk in light of projected benefits.

Thorough cost/benefit weighing also requires, albeit less easily and precisely, the balancing of subjective features of the new conceptions. Because so much of expanded IVF means using techniques that have infrequently been tried and for which little data are available, subjective factors are often all that are available.

One commonly feared cost said to be paired with IVF is the diminishing of humanness. Leon Kass feels that the costs of IVF and genetic engineering to the family are too great to justify the benefits. He writes:

"The family is rapidly becoming the only institution in an increasingly impersonal world where each person is loved not for what he does nor makes, but simply because he is."[32] Paul Ramsey thought IVF contributes to the "manufactury of children" and Kass argues that it turns attention to the "products" of conception manufactured under the "bright (fluorescent) light of the laboratory."[33]

New conceptions are also said to degrade embryos, women, men and unborn children. The more variations, it is argued, the more is the embryo manipulated and graded; the family subdivided into genetic, gestational, and legal parents; the romance of conception pummeled; and women and men valued for their ability to produce sperm, eggs, and uteruses. Men produce sperm for Nobel prize sperm banks; the act of producing sperm by masturbation is in itself degrading.[34] New conceptions degrade marriage by separating procreation from the sexual act:

Test tube babies are "in nature" but not "according to nature" since their procreation is not united to the conjugal act.[35]

Human procreation is begetting. It . . . engages us bodily and spiritually, as well as rationally. . . . Before embarking on New Beginnings in Life we should consider the meaning of the union between sex, love and procreation, and the meaning and consequence of its cleavage.[36]

New conceptions are said to pose hidden costs of powerlessness on the women who use them. According to founders of the Feminist International Network of Resistance to Reproductive and Genetic Engineering (FINRRAGE), which was formed in 1984, the new conceptions are an effort by "misogynous science" to make profits from and experiment on women.[37] It is thought that the technology "insults and degrades" women under the guise of helping them.[38] Among other things, IVF raises the prospects of gender selection and a preponderance of men over women; a felt responsibility by women to have healthy babies; and increasing mechanization of childbearing.[39] When IVF is done with donated ova and embryos, female reproduction is dissected in a way that downgrades women's power and magnifies control over reproduction by men.[40]

Margaret Atwood captures fictionally the ultimate use of women for their bodies in *The Handmaid's Tale* where, in the future state of Gilead, plummeting Caucasian birthrates turn women into reproducers. As the nameless handmaid narrator says, "We are two-legged wombs, that's all:

sacred vessels, ambulatory chalices." This handmaid had once, before the Gilead government was set up, thought of her body as a whole— "lithe, single, solid, one with me." After months as an intended receptacle for fertilization and birth, she now thinks of herself as an object. Her identity has become one with her uterus: "Now the flesh arranges itself differently. I'm a cloud, congealed around a central object, the shape of a pear, which is hard and more real than I am and glows red within its translucent wrapping."[41]

Assault to the dignity of the embryo is another subjective cost argued especially by those who act as spiritual attorneys for the embryo, representing it and attesting to its inherent value.[42] One geneticist, for example, contends that when the 23 chromosomes from the female and the 23 chromosomes from the male meet, "the full genetic information, necessary and sufficient to spell out all the inborn qualities of the new individual, is gathered:"

Exactly as the introduction of a minicassette inside a tape recorder will allow the "re-creation" of the symphony, the information included in the 46 chromosomes (the minicassettes of the symphony of life) will be deciphered by the machinery of the cytoplasm of the fertilized egg (the tape recorder), and the new being begins to express himself as soon as he has been conceived.[43]

At the point of fertilization, "a unique potential member of our species is created."[44] Although the embryo "cannot inquire, understand, read or write," this is not important; neither can babies, some handicapped persons, comatose people, or even sleeping persons.[45] All, however, have rights as humans; the human embryo is "a fellow human being and, as a consequence, worthy of all the protection we afford ourselves."[46] It is thought that IVF negates that protection.

The new conceptions also are said to produce subjective benefits for individuals and society. Some suggest that far from dehumanizing us, when we use technology we are at our most intrinsically human and to use technology to create a family is one of the more human endeavors of all.[47] New conceptions in this line of thinking are no more dehumanizing than using an incubator for a premature infant or performing a caesarean section for a troublesome birth.[48] What is dehumanizing to the couple is not IVF but instead the isolated struggle to conceive when couples are infertile but have nowhere to turn. As for the embryo, a common view is that the embryo is not a human and if some are lost in order for a conception to take place, this is an insignificant loss. The benefit coming from one child outweighs the cost resulting from the loss of dozens or hundreds of embryos.

An Ethic of Choice: A Summary. Neither moral reasoning nor cost/benefit thinking alone is sufficient for developing patterns of individual choice when faced with the cafeteria of reproductive choice. Instead, the pairing of the empirical with the emotional, the objective with the subjective, and the absolute with the relative together will be used by individuals depending on their preferences and background. The precise "recipe" is less important than the message that comes from the quest for guidance: there is a choice and there are criteria for reaching that choice. Consumption must be circumspect; the quest for guiding principles in itself conveys the message that limits are appropriate.

A RESPONSIBLE PUBLIC

Anna Quindlen, a newspaper columnist, pondered the Baby M case and asked what she would have done had she and her husband not been able to have children: "If I had not been able to give birth to my children as I did, I would have done anything to get them—place ads; pay money; maybe, just maybe, hire someone to give birth to them for us. Anything. Anything at all."[49]

The fact that she could see a range of options is indicative of great changes that have taken place in the last two decades. Egg donation, embryo donation, and surrogacy, as innovations peculiar to the 1980s, and the prospect of genetic manipulations in the 1990s have prompted thinking about choice and created a need to find standards to guide these choices. One IVF clinician expressed impatience at commentators who paired IVF with such issues as surrogacy: "it is only logical that a discussion of the ethics of in-vitro fertilization be confined to a discussion of the ethics of in-vitro fertilization."[50] Yet events revolving around expanded IVF tell us we need to understand the values we hold in order to understand our role as consumers of individual techniques.

The ballad "I Am My Own Grandpa" swept in and out of the music lexicon in the early twentieth century. In it the singer marries his step-grandmother and now wonders who he was supposed to call granddad. The song records his lament as he realizes his plight: he is his own grandpa. This ballad could very well have been written in the 1980s when a child using her mother's egg and her father's sperm could sing, if she had a daughter, "I Am My Sister's Mother" or the mother could sing her own ballad, "My Daughter Is My Daughter's Mother," or the child could croon, "My Mother Is My Sister."[51] The new techniques force us to think of such things that were once merely fanciful.

In orienting the discussion, there are things we can do as responsible citizens. We are not mere spectators but are instead potential consumers and the progenitors of tomorrow's users of new conceptions. What role can we play in developing an ethic of choice?

Closing the Distance. One thing we can do is try to get closer to the reality of IVF. In this we would go against a pattern of distancing that has marked public reaction to IVF. Jonathan Glover writes that we suffer a "paralysis of the imagination" when we distance ourselves from an event. When observing from a distance we lose focus of that which we are witnessing and, with it, we lose focus of what we can do about the event.[52] The early parties to IVF—physicians, scientists, journalists, ethicists, policymakers, and patients—all used symbols and beliefs that built a distance between IVF and their own responsibility for it.

Physicians distanced themselves by looking at the ends (successful pregnancies) while skimming over the means (the hopes and feelings of the couples who were the IVF pioneers). They "telescoped" to the end of quantifiable goals and, if the writings of early IVF practitioners are an indication, tended to skip over the everyday costs to patients incurred by the experimentation. To illustrate, when reporting on the first IVF pregnancy, prematurely ended because it was ectopic, Edwards and Steptoe wrote that as a result surgery was needed to remove the woman's right fallopian tube as well as her "diseased left tube." The report gives little indication of the costs to the woman, however, in terms of her now double tube failure and the inconvenience of surgery. Instead, the authors wrote that "the patient made a rapid recovery and was discharged from the hospital a week later."[53] The editors of the journal in which the report was published added an unusual postscript: "I am sure that everyone wishes the investigators well in this very difficult area of experimentation."

Physicians distance themselves with the language of coolness in the medicine of IVF and, as the freezing experience suggests, in the social implications of IVF, with talk of disposition of property, ownership, disposal, and other terms normally used for nonliving objects. Physicians and laypersons alike have tried to figure out what to call expanded IVF itself, with possibilities including "noncoital reproduction," "external human fertilization," "assisted conception," "new conceptions," and "human assisted reproduction."[54]

Patients distance themselves when they say "no amount of pain is too much," they are "desperate," or they are "willing to try anything" to conceive. Such talk divorces them from the consequences of their actions and diminishes their role as participants in decision making. They create their own slippery slope when they suggest they have no control over the course of their action and are propelled by IVF as the last chance and by ticking biological clocks. They telescope to the future when they look more for an answer to infertility than to a pregnancy itself. They distance themselves with a language of depersonalism when they measure and evaluate themselves on the size and number of their follicles and the number and quality of their eggs and embryos.

For ethicists and scholarly observers, the slippery slope is a distancing mechanism that suggests humans cannot be responsible once technology gains momentum. Their talk of artificiality, baby making, and production spreads the very image of artificiality and does little to enhance public understanding of the clinical practice of IVF.[55] Policymakers distance themselves by pairing IVF with abortion and genetic engineering and concluding that IVF is a "hot," "sticky," and "touchy" issue. Journalists distance themselves with labels of test-tube baby, test-tube mother, baby in a bottle, baby from the lab, and, with freezing, deep frozen test-tube baby.[56]

All of this makes more distant our feelings of responsibility for new conceptions. If the world of reproductive techniques is a world in which objects are produced, we have created a "we-they" distinction and allow ourselves to bow out of the arena. It is small wonder that one woman pregnant through IVF told an acquaintance she was going to her physician for a checkup and was asked in response, "What do they do? Check the tube?" The misconceptions bred by inaccurate imagery engender the feeling of "Who me? I have nothing to do with *that.*"

As citizens, we can heighten our feelings of control and responsibility by being vigilant about the imagery coming to us from different quarters. Test-tube babydom is an idiosyncratic image in an era of artificial organs and techniques. We do not talk about "dialysis men" or "valve women" or "pacemaker persons" or use other labels that marry people to techniques. We do not call premature infants "incubated tots" or those born by caesarean section "scalpel youngsters." On the contrary, if we equate a person's identity with medical treatments, we run the risk of unsettling prejudice as, for example, calling a man with an artificial leg "peg-leg Pete."

To be progressive in the 1980s is to use prepositions (e.g., a person who is blind) rather than adjectives (a blind person) when referring to a person's attributes in order to avoid pairing a person's identity with his or her physical features.[57] In the area of IVF, however, the adjectives are alive and well. In fact, the pairing of attribute with identity threatens to grow with expanded IVF. In one cartoon a woman looks down at a puddle of water on the sidewalk. On top of the puddle lies a baseball cap. "It happens on hot days," she explains to her friend. "Johnny was a frozen embryo."[58] Another cartoon shows a chauffeur holding open a limousine door as a penguin steps out. One bystander says knowingly to another, "I understand he inherited a fortune when he was a frozen embryo."[59]

One wonders if the reaction to IVF would be different if we used terms that did not divorce embryos and children of the new conceptions symbolically from the rest of humanity. In the absence of data indicating children conceived externally are any different from other babies, one wonders if it serves any purpose to call them anything. Images set in a context of humanness will arguably set in motion a more empathic view of IVF and in so doing help us appreciate our responsibilities as citizens. The suggestion of humanizing embryos comes at some risk, however. Right-to-life groups are only too eager to call embryos and fetuses "babies" in order to prevent IVF. The intention here is, on the contrary, to create a bond between the public and IVF by speaking a language that will help overcome the we-they distinction in public discussions of IVF. In vitro fertilization is not something done in back rooms to objects. It is a process involving the beginnings of an infant's life, and we as individuals who want to protect this matter must regard it with sensitivity.

Desperation, slopes, test-tube babies, miracles, and property all discourage insight into that which is homely and human in a technique many prefer to call science fiction. What passes as a miracle cure for desperate patients and a window for the brightest minds is, when stripped of its theatrical wrappings, little more than a simple medical transaction. Denuded of flamboyancy, basic IVF with fresh tissues and married couples is a rather simple buying and selling exchange. Physicians offer IVF for couples with a particular need. Thus, as a responsible public, we can wrest control of the imagery and create our own more realistic, less distant interpretation of new conceptions.

Self-Knowledge About Our Anxieties. In general, we greet technology amiably and we invite symbols of that technology into our popular culture, with Hal, the talking computer; Robocop, the "half man/half machine"; R2-D2; and Buck Rogers part of that legend. We embrace technology as something that pushes our land into modernity and we see modernity as a positive "condition that there can be indefinite progress because there is always something new and better to find."[60] The National Air and Space Museum in Washington is testimony to our spirit of exploration; in it people throng to see the moonlanding module, Amelia Earhart's flaming red plane, and the sleek, cigar-winged *Voyager*.

With IVF and its promise of exploration inside the human embryo we felt malaise, fueled by fervent headlines, dire warnings, and literary allusions. Prometheus, Faust, Sisyphus, and Frankenstein all joined the public debate. There would be no museum commemorating the first union of ovum and sperm in a glass dish. This event was not the sort that shot John Glenn straight up in space and right back down. This nascent biotechnology was thought to portend open genie bottles with unsettling consequences.

Uncertainty has pulsed through the history of IVF and is expressed in the form of dark humor, a not uncommon reaction to anxiety. In one comic strip, a writer works at his typewriter. "Mary had a little lamb," he begins. He pauses, thinks, and finishes the story. "And so she sued the test-tube baby laboratory."[61] A political cartoon shows a scientist watching faceless, T-shirted humanoids wandering around a factory room. "For the last time, Fudsworth," he complains to the factory lineman, "It is genetic engineering, not *generic* engineering I wanted."[62] The humor cloaks basic fears. *Would* humans be mass produced? What *will* the children be like?

Why is there this uncertainty in reaction to a single technological event? Perhaps *Brave New World* had primed us with its story of a fictionalized setting that paired test-tube fertilization with a total loss of autonomy and individuality. Yet *Brave New World* did not create fears; rather, it built on nightmarish visions lively before the book was written during Stalin's "socialism in one country" and at the onset of Hitler's Third Reich. Huxley himself felt fear. About his society of decanters, predestinators, and Alphas, Betas, and Gammas, he wrote: "We are getting more and more in a position where these things can be achieved. And it's extremely important to realize this, and to take every precaution to see that they shall *not* be achieved. This, I take it was the message of the book—*This is possible: for heaven's sake be careful about it.*"[63]

Part of our malaise undoubtedly relates to feared loss of control. We use the "smoke-filled room" to symbolize our distrust of an elite group of political figures making decisions secretly and for their own advantage. Similarly, our image of the "white-coated laboratory scientist" tells of our distrust about what scientists are doing without our knowledge and for their own arcane purpose. Gena Corea, thinking about Edwards' experiments using eggs from women having ovarectomies, wrote of the omnipotent and depersonalized scientist:

When the women consented to the surgery, did they know that as they lay anesthesized on the table, a man would be standing there waiting to collect their eggs in a glass pot? Did they know that, in at least one instance in Cambridge, he would add his sperm to their eggs in an attempt at fertilization in a dish? Did they ever dream of eggs—their own eggs—fertilized by a *faceless man in a white laboratory coat?*"[64]

Amitai Etzioni, author of *The Genetic Fix*, entitled one of his chapters, "An Overview: What Are *They* Brewing For Us?" and a British columnist asked, "How are [members of Parliament] to know what geneticists do in the *dark watches of the night?*"[65] These questions convey a sense of fatalism in the face of scientific expertise and a worry that isolated scientists, bereft of human compassion, will carry out experiments un-impeded, unmanaged, secretively, and scurrilously: "Dr Faustus, Dr Frankenstein, Dr Moreau, Dr Jekyll, Dr Cyclops, Dr Caligari, Dr Strangelove . . . In these images of our popular culture resides a legiti-mate public fear of the scientist's ripped down, depersonalized concep-tion of knowledge—a fear that our scientists will go on being titans who create monsters."[66]

We also nurse the hope that some things—including conception—will be left "shrouded in mystery."[67] In vitro fertilization denies us that mystery and reveals conception in its minute detail: the egg's jelly-like cumulus, the spermatozoan's grip as it enters the egg, the waving tails of the sperm that fail to enter waving on the egg's perimeter like delicate fuzz, the grainy-appearing interior of the cleaving cells, and even the shrunken, raisin-like look of the embryo that stops cleaving. No longer a mystery, conception becomes predictable, controllable, scientific, and even, think some, superior to the hostile conditions of natural concep-tion.[68] To explain conception threatens to deprive us of one measure of humanness—our intrigue with the unknown.

Surely a part of the underlying anxiety about IVF is traceable to fears we will be abandoned by the opposite sex. Two possibilities that evoke concern—asexual reproduction and the artificial womb—each would make one gender dispensable. With the former, an egg cell can be taken from a woman, split, and united with another body cell, rendering the male superfluous. With the latter, the woman becomes a mere provider of eggs and she, too, is rendered superfluous. Will women and men, no longer needing one another to perpetuate their species, abandon the other? Would August Strindberg's recommendation come true?

> Woman, being small and foolish and therefore evil . . . should be suppressed, like barbarians and thieves. She is useful only as ovary and womb. . . . She can be replaced, dispensed with. One needs only a constant temperature of 37° and a suitable nourishment fluid. Then man will be emancipated.[69]

Our malaise may also be due in part to a need to assert control over something concrete in an era in which we are capable of destroying ourselves through nuclear war. If we feel powerless about nuclear armament, perhaps we can protect embryos as the tiniest among us. The tendency to focus on that which is close is a trait of human nature. When we cannot comprehend a multi-billion dollar national budget, our policymakers fight over programs costing mere tens of thousands of dollars. When a "child down the road gets drowned," we care more "than if thousands die in a flood in another country." We "take a more charitable view of others who kill at at distance than those who do at close range."[70] Moral outrage over what is done to embryos is a way of wresting control over something tangible.

There may even be a conceit at work in our reaction to IVF. When someone claims that the recombination of human genes is "the most important and disturbing technological change in recorded history,"[71] we must wonder if the claim has a touch of puffery to it that signals a masked pride in being part of a singular era.

Or perhaps our reaction is partly the work of our imaginative minds flirting with morbid but safely distant visions. We sashay with apocalypse, and "we like to make our flesh creep, though not to the point where our flesh actually stings."[72] Maybe predictions of "neo-Hitlers" and "throngs of dustmen" are our way of flirting with goblins, in the same way listeners readily believed Orson Wells' radiocast of the "War of the Worlds" or happily wait in line to see the "thriller of the decade." Predicting the worst is for the most part safe. Our history demonstrates that, for the most part, new technologies just make life more comfortable.

In vitro fertilization is, in short, a symptom as well as a cause of anxiety. As responsible citizens we must take care that IVF not become the whipping boy for other, more deeply rooted anxieties. Not only does misdirected anxiety place a burden on IVF as victim, but it prevents us from facing our anxieties and finding effective ways of dealing with them.

An Attitude of Control. We also can work to develop an attitude of control over that which causes anxiety. This means demystifying the technique. It also means resisting the temptation to hide behind the cloak of the so-called technological imperative (what can be done will be done; if we don't do it someone else will). In 1987 *Harper's Magazine* brought together a panel of experts to debate issues posed by genetic technologies. Jeremy Rifkin, a vocal critic of reproductive technologies, predicted future excesses and downward spirals, while two ethicists presented a more positive counterpoint. Eventually, after Rifkin pointed to negative futures perhaps once too often, one of the panel members, Nancy Dubler, blurted, "Again, Jeremy, you hold no faith in our ability to make any distinctions, any reasonable judgments." Herein lay the thorn. Critics such as Rifkin who appear to negate our ability to control technology, stray from the norm of faith in the ability of Americans to limit themselves. "We can draw lines," one of the panelists said. "We are human beings; we deal with difficult problems all the time." [73]

An attitude of control will grow from our willingness to look at our achievements in placing limits. The ideology we build must do more than lament the rapidity of change; it must also highlight ways in which we have slowed the pace of change by deliberate policy. For whatever problems the disbanding of the EAB has posed, the act itself is significant as an example of imposing limits. As Leon R. Kass observes: "Perhaps for the first time in the modern era of biomedical research, public deliberation and debate about ethical matters led to an effective moratorium on Federal support for experimentation—in this case, for research on human *in vitro* fertilization. [74]

We can point to studies showing there are options patients will *not* take. [75] We can look at agreement on what should be limited in the new conceptions reached by members of commissions on new conceptions set up by the hundreds around the world. [76] We can look at the commissions themselves as evidence that persons in Western democracies want to entertain limits. We can look to policies, however rough, enacted or attempted by governments trying to limit new conceptions in Australia, Britain, Germany, and elsewhere. [77] We can see efforts by the U.S. government to limit recombinant DNA research.

In 1933 Chicagoans welcomed the World's Fair with the theme "Science Finds—Industry Applies—Man Conforms." Dorothy Nelkin wonders what that theme would be if rewritten today. She suggests it might more appropriately be "Science Finds—Industry Applies—Man Controls." [78] When a technology provokes as great an outcry as did IVF, it is essential for us to build an ideology of confidence that reflects our ability to limit the pace and breadth of that technology. This involves confronting our anxieties, asserting control over the images of high-tech medicine, and building successful limits into our behavior on the basis of ethical or other predetermined criteria.

CHAPTER SEVEN

Looking to the Future

W hen I was a child a neighbor, four years older and surely knowledgeable about such matters, told me that the square brown UPS delivery trucks combed the streets looking for children to take away. How large the truck loomed in my mind as I dived into the bushes every time I saw one coming. What resistance could I, a child with arms and legs the width of batons, offer to the giant of a truck that seemed to grow exponentially every time it lumbered down the street? The trucks stood in my mind as evil personified.

The world of IVF contains within it some of the more colorful behemoths in modern-day technology. Early warnings of unparalleled sweeps down a slippery slope to negative consequences captured our attention just as surely as would warnings of child-snatching for children on city streets. These warnings implanted an unsettling doubt in our ability to manage and direct the new reproductive technologies. Even though the most sensationalistic warnings have waned with IVF's largely humdrum medical practice, doubts linger about our ability to initiate policy and set limits on new and provocative applications of assisted conception.

The preceding chapters have argued that our record of management is stronger than often believed. Daniel Callahan writes that "As a society, we do not know what to do with technological advances that promise both benefit and harm. . . . We must devise almost *de novo* a methodology and decision-making procedure." [1] This methodology will have new elements, to be sure, but it will be grounded on achievements already reached. To build a policy of expanded IVF that will accompany us into the twenty-first century we need to use the success we have already reached. More importantly, we must expect and encourage responsible consumption by the parties to IVF and by ourselves as the parents of tomorrow's consumers. Neither elaborate legislation nor elaborate consumption is appropriate at this time. Instead, we need to move slowly, cautiously, and with confidence as we shed self-defeating ideas of slippery slopes and technological imperatives and turn to the human and manageable dimensions of expanded IVF.

CHALLENGING PREVAILING MYTHS AND SYMBOLS

S ymbols, myths, and metaphors reflect today's beliefs and shape tomorrow's ideas.[2] George Orwell has written of the "huge dump of worn-out metaphors which have lost all evocative power and are merely used because they save people the trouble of inventing phrases for themselves."[3] Our approach to new conceptions must go hand in hand with constant testing of symbols and language. The colorful symbols of test-tube babies, manufactured children, cloned hominids, and the Brave New World are now being replaced by less colorful but equally significant symbols of desperate patients, infertility epidemic, embryos as property, IVF as a window, and embryo research as a vehicle.

In the first ten years of IVF the persons who have initiated prevailing symbols have changed from largely nonmedical critics to mainly medical proponents, with a corresponding shift in the direction of the prevailing metaphor. No longer is IVF seen as the first step down a slope of horrors, but it is depicted as the first step up a ladder of beneficial applications. This ideology warrants challenge just as surely as did the ideology before it. In fact, the IVF as "up" metaphor arguably warrants even closer scrutiny because it has come quietly and with the authority of the medical profession behind it. It presumes IVF's benefits to society, yet decisions about what resources to allocate to research and clinical applications of expanded IVF have not yet been widely debated. Symbols that invite affirmative policy are as important to scrutinize as are symbols warning of the need for controls.

BUILDING FROM CONSENSUS

T he great majority of citizens favor basic IVF, and virtually all commission reports here and abroad conclude that IVF is ethically acceptable. The consensus about using a wife's and husband's gametes for external fertilization to produce an embryo when the couple is infertile has been here from the start, diverted by small groups of detractors. The overwhelming public value is that couples who want a child but cannot have one should have access to a technique that can help them. Other points of consensus, garnered from commission reports, the EAB report, interest group statements, and from occasional public opinion polls, are that: IVF must be administered humanely, expanded IVF must be introduced cautiously, in a crisis the child's interests outweigh the couple's interests, clinical applications that would change the nature of being human (e.g., genetic applications) are to be treated with special scrutiny, physicians are basically trustworthy, procreation is a private matter, and debate and discussion are appropriate.

A presumption of permissiveness pervades these points of agreement. This is promising because we can start policy from a half-full glass; it is troubling because it indicates the attitudinal changes toward circumspect consumption advocated in this book will not come easily. On the contrary, the burden of proof will lie with those who want to limit research, development, and consumption. Still, the points of agreement tell us we should develop a policy with authority shared by private and public sectors. Despite lingering fears of "white-coated scientists," there is among the public and policymakers a trust in the goodness of science and a skepticism of the ability of legislators to make policy relating to reproductive technologies. A *de novo* methodology will respect the existing partnership between IVF practitioners and public decision makers.

BUILDING INCREMENTALLY

O liver Wendell Holmes once surmised that "The life of the law has not been logic; it has been experience."[4] Our shaky confidence in our ability to manage reproductive technologies is largely due to early attempts to define the issue in futuristic terms for which we had no skills to deal. Predicted negative outcomes motivated us to act but gave no help for that action. The law is at its most useful when grounded in everyday experience and observation. Although anticipating problems is a critical element in policymaking, anticipation must be counterbalanced with factual experience.

The method adopted in this book has been to take as a starting point for policy the daily behavior of the physicians, scientists, and patients most intimately involved with IVF. By examining the "goodness" with which IVF is administered in the private sector, we can erect a starting point for building a policy of IVF. To see what practitioners have done in the absence of governmental oversight is to give a blueprint for deciding what policy is appropriate and what can be left to private sector initiative. Observed deficiencies in hospital and professional group guidelines help identify policy needs that ought to be addressed by governments. In other cases, hospital policies are so well developed they can serve as models for later public policy or as substitutes for that policy. Several conclusions can be drawn.

First, practitioners are relatively effective at monitoring quality control in the clinical application of IVF. The power of the marketplace, protectiveness about the field of infertility, distrust of government "meddling," institutional pride, and the fear of lawsuits all create incentives for practitioners to be cautious about new medical protocols. These incentives are arguably as effective as regulatory controls. Medical interest groups thus should be encouraged to continue self-policing activities and to participate in public hearings and meetings about the application of IVF. The models for achieving quality control developed in the private sector can be used in later policy as, for example, the Maryland law that provides for the insurance reimbursement of IVF only for patients who go to clinics conforming to AFS and ACOG standards.

Second, practitioners are less perceptive about "goodness" in the nonmedical aspects of IVF protocol. When it comes to sensitivity about the emotional components of IVF and about fair warning to patients of success rates and risks of new techniques, practitioners have fewer incentives to police themselves; in fact, they may have a greater incentive to dissemble and present a more glowing picture than warranted in order to draw patients and test IVF variations.

As an injustice, the lack of adequate information to patients is not a topic for new legislation, however. Deficiencies in truth in packaging and the context for informed consent can be addressed by existing malpractice, commerce, and medical codes. The apparatus for addressing injustices is already in place; the remedy is not to set up new laws but instead to encourage publicity about ills, educate consumers about injustices and remedies, and counteract symbols of IVF as the last and only hope that discourage patients from drawing negative attention to the way IVF is administered. One patient wrote of the frustration of being indebted to doctors for IVF treatment:

We, as patients, are not in a position to comment objectively about many IVF issues . . . For most couples our dearest wish is to have a child so we do not publicly complain about the endless experimental procedures, the dehumanised method of treatment, the pain, cost and emotional strain that is an integral part of IVF. I have known some to complain but only to incur the wrath of the IVF team.[5]

Before laws are passed, efforts must be made to encourage patients and potential patients openly to discuss the weaknesses and strengths of everyday IVF practice.

Third, practitioners lack logical, agreed-upon, and consistent criteria in deciding how to administer variations of IVF. The earliest policy is being framed in IVF clinics and the basis of that policy, if we use embryo freezing as a case study, is based on expediency, trial and error, and blind modeling across centers. Incorrect or hurtful policies are copied from center to center like a ditto machine gone awry. Again, this inappropriate behavior should not be remedied through legislation but, rather, by education, publicity, and cross-disciplinary involvement (e.g., through ethics committees) when IVF variations are set up. It is a fact of the medical world that doctors tend to filter issues to the level of medical protocol and clinical judgment.[6] They cannot necessarily be faulted for skimming over moral dilemmas when setting up IVF programs but they can be faulted for not recognizing the moral component and for not setting up a process of inviting nonmedical points of view into decision making.

It is judicious to set up ethics committees, get written feedback from patients about improving their programs, invite nurse coordinators and outside consultants to speak out at staff meetings, and take other steps to meet the societal obligation of administering new conceptions with care and sensitivity. This can also be achieved through persistent pressure from patients, women's interest groups, medical consumer groups, ethicists, and others willing to find out what is going on and to talk about it.

In summary, we need to look at experience before building policy in order to see injustices that can be remedied by existing auxilliary mechanisms, and we need to encourage publicity about those injustices. It is important not to be waylaid by the quest to develop elaborate public policy when some rather simple mechanisms will suffice. The issue ought to be how to gather data about the administration of IVF's variations, publicize injustices, encourage an even-handed review of ongoing medical practices that is not unnecessarily apologetic or condemnatory, reduce the vulnerability patients feel about complaining about IVF treatment, and push for a rational system for reaching medical decisions about IVF. The government's role in building a policy of IVF must therefore be, first of all, to set up forums for investigation and analysis. These forums can take the form of public reports (e.g., the report on infertility issued by the Office of Technology Assessment), Congressional hearings, executive agencies that contract with medical groups to gather data about IVF practice, and grants for model programs of the administration of new conceptions.

There are many advantages to an incremental approach based on experience and observation. Incrementalism encourages us to address actual problems facing medical patients now; encourage responsibility by those who initiate and practice IVF; help us as citizens to build a track record of success in stimulating behavioral changes in the clinical setting; and set the stage for the daily management of new techniques. It is a matter of recycling and energizing existing policy before tinkering with new policy. Indiscriminant consumption of policy (do something—pass any law—now) is no more acceptable than indiscriminant consumption of sophisticated techniques.

ASSERTING INDIVIDUAL RESPONSIBILITY

Hans Jonas has said of new technologies that they "suggest, create, even impose ends never thought of before, simply by offering their feasibility."[7] Technology is seductive. It ensnares us by posing solutions to things we did not know were problems and it offers the glamor of the hunt for those solutions.

Scientific inquiry takes on a meaning in itself. Those engaged in scientific discovery occasionally experience "a rare kind of exhilaration that Socrates said was the greatest of human pleasures."[8] Finding answers to problems also takes on a meaning in itself, as in the people whose "dearest wish" is to have a child and who try first one then another enticement for achieving that wish. To put brakes on scientific discovery and clinical applications goes against the grain of deeply held beliefs in Western culture. Yet seduction deprives persons of the free and enlightened exercise of their will. Created needs create victims. The purer satisfaction of technology comes from the ability freely to discriminate between actual and created needs and between pressure and spontaneous wishes to consume. To assert our will in the context of mounting pressure to use reproductive technologies, we as individuals must be wary of the trap of unlimited consumption and be prepared to assert limits on that consumption.

For physicians this means searching for authentic reasons for offering variations of IVF based on service to the patient rather than professional advancement or inter-clinic competition. It also means enlarging and examining the concept of "service" to ask: does this protocol serve the emotional needs of the patient? does this protocol create a need that did not previously exist? A discriminating physician will offer variations only after sufficient data exist to inform the patient of the odds of success and of the benefits and costs. Physicians engaged in research on IVF variations (e.g., egg freezing) will clearly convey this to the patient and consider not charging the patient for the procedure.

Discriminating physicians will develop a thoughtful way of adding new procedures to the clinic. Physicians unwilling to do this ought to wait until suggested procedures have been reached by interest groups such as the American Fertility Society. They will also be sensitive to the societal implications of how they offer new techniques and, following the counsel of Edmund Pellegrino, will be attuned to the ethical criteria to which they personally refer when making decisions about patients.[9] The discriminating physician will give full information about the successes and failures of IVF variations at his or her clinic. Physicians who feel the need to dissemble and distort success rates or use global rates can take this as a sign that their clinic is not ready to be offering the variation.

The most obvious way patients can assert individual responsibility is to decline to participate in experimental protocols that offer low odds of success and unknown risks but for which clinics charge fees. The principle will carry over even if insurance covers the charges; the idea of charging for highly experimental protocols places patients in the role of victims and perpetuates a system in which physicians offer new techniques as a way of bringing income to their clinics. For couples determined to try whatever it takes, no matter what the odds, their responsibility is to ask questions, challenge the physician, and let it be known they expect comprehensive information. Patients will also freely discuss their experiences in order to help build appropriate and sensitive protocols in IVF centers. The successes of IVF ought to reduce protectiveness toward the procedure; IVF is no longer vulnerable to being banned. Criticism will help, not hinder, its operations.

National legislators can take on individual responsibility by addressing issues surrounding IVF for infertile women before moving to new, perhaps more politically exciting fields, such as help for veterans with service-related infertility or the allocation of funds for embryo research geared to understanding and preventing genetic diseases. Responsible policymakers will also welcome debate about new conceptions, set up forums for the debate, and be wary about prematurely placing public resources behind expanded IVF. Affirmative policy ought to be built slowly with insight about the limitations to be imposed (is it to help infertile couples? all infertile couples? will infertility be a health care priority? should IVF be used to circumvent genetic defects? is it more important to allocate funds for this than for infertility?). Legislators will also encourage policy experimentation at the state level and carry out follow-up studies of different policy models before enacting national policy.

BUILDING A LANGUAGE OF CONTROL

It is not enough simply to assert individual limits; we also need to build a language that embraces an *expectation* we can manage new conceptions. First we must develop the habit of talking about applications that will not do. At present, for example, ethics commissions here and abroad suggest research not be done on embryos beyond fourteen days after fertilization. This is a reasonable (if arbitrary) recommendation and does not penalize researchers—embryos have not been kept alive that long and there are few specific ideas about what would be done with fourteen-day-old embryos in any event. Still, though, some commentators complain about the limit, saying it is all right for now but should be open to change or saying the limit should be extended to fifty days or longer.[10] This limit has value as a symbol of our ability to draw lines, however. No matter what its faults, it conveys the important message that persons of different disciplines around the world have agreed that research on human embryos beyond fourteen days will not, at present, do.

After certain applications are excluded from consideration in this manner, we are left with a range of possibilities that may or may not be acceptable. With these possibilities, we need to develop a language of evaluation that becomes part of our vocabulary and conveys the expectation of management. As suggested in earlier chapters, this might take the form of clear and present danger and benefit tests. It is not enough simply to assert that a technique will help couples. Before resources are distributed, we need to ask and receive assurances that it is highly likely in the immediate future clearly to benefit a specific group of persons. The criteria of proximity and degree are valid tools for scientists in the laboratory, physicians in the clinic, and legislators in the statehouse. Always the questions must be asked: who will benefit? precisely how will they benefit? when will they benefit? is it important that they benefit?

CONCLUSION

There is much that can be done as we move from laboratories to legislatures. We can question the new routines coming from IVF centers. We can narrow the questions asked in order to invigorate the debate. We can put a human face on IVF by talking with patients and doctors to find out what is going on in clinics and to make this information accessible to lay citizens. We can root out dead metaphors and language and we can ask who is being harmed by their continuation. By our revulsion about certain applications, we can specify what will not do. We can frame questions in ways that are politically useful for our culture by making them empirical, present-oriented, and incremental. We can seek to develop an expectation of control. Above all, we can slow the pace. If we cannot stop the march of technology, we can at least pause to wonder, "what is the rush?"

The first decade of IVF was one of mobilizing attention and setting the blueprint in broad strokes. The second decade is the time for laying the foundation and building, step by step, from there. Creativity has played its role. The time for incremental work is here. We must gather information, question the ends being sought, and use our insight as a beacon for enlightened management of beckoning techniques.

When confronted by his department chair in 1973 with the vial containing the Del Zios' sperm and eggs, the supervising physician suggested, "Let me just throw this thing out, okay?" to which his chair replied, "Leave it here, no, please." [11] Many discoveries loom in the field of reproductive medicine that have more to do with human needs than with the technology itself. For a true understanding of basic IVF, we would be wise to "leave it here, please" long enough to ponder our responses so far. We would be irresponsible to move further into expanded IVF before appreciating the human side of basic IVF and building confidence in our ability to pause and manage as yet unknown applications one step at a time.

The IVF Technique

The IVF medical protocol takes approximately two weeks and includes the stages of ovulation induction, egg retrieval, fertilization, and embryo transfer. During ovulation induction, the woman takes a combination of hormones to stimulate her ovaries and her body "reacts abnormally, producing two, three, four or more eggs."[1] During the days she receives the medication, she is monitored by blood draws and ultrasonography to make sure her follicles are responding. Physicians measure this response by the estradiol level of the blood and the number and size of follicles.

Centers generally want to see two or three follicles 3 centimeters in diameter (approximately 1-¼") before operating to drain the follicles.[2] Technicians view the follicles through the abdominal wall by ultrasound for each of several days before the expected surgery. To prepare for ultrasonography, the woman drinks at least 30 ounces of liquid 45 minutes before the scheduled ultrasound (translated into "recipes" by patients who repeatedly undergo ultrasounds, such as the woman who drinks two 4½ ounce cans of orange juice, one pint of orange juice, one 12-ounce Tab, and three 16-ounce cups of water). The liquid creates a full bladder which pushes the bowel out of the way for a better view of the ovaries. Technicians rub a blue gel on the stomach and move a transducer across it to show the follicles on the screen.

When monitoring runs smoothly, human chorionic gonadotrophin (HCG) is injected to simulate a hormonal surge, indicate that ovulation will take place approximately 36 hours later, and precisely time the eggs' ripening.

The HCG is usually given in the evening so the surgery can be scheduled for the morning, 36 hours later, right before the anticipated release of eggs from the follicles. The goal is to time the laparoscopy to occur just before the eggs are released but after they have reached a stage of maturation known as metaphase II that signals their ripeness for fertilization. The practitioner's ability to control the timing of the surge and surgery has improved since IVF's early years when operations took place at all hours and monitoring was less precise. Then women had to take frequent urine samples to detect the luteinizing hormone (LH) surge and they had blood draws up to four times a day.[3]

Eggs are retrieved most commonly in a surgery known as the laparoscopy. The operation is done under a light general anesthetic to protect the eggs. The woman is generally awake when her stomach is scrubbed and may even have walked into the operating chamber. During the laparoscopy, surgeons make two or three short, ½ inch incisions in the abdomen. They insert a forceps into one incision in the abdomen. They insert a forceps into one incision to locate the ovaries, hold them still, and move adhesions aside if they block the way to the ovaries.[4] They insert a hollow needle through which the follicular fluid will be suctioned into the second incision. The needle is lined with teflon, which has "the lowest surface friction of any material known," so the fluid and eggs will not attach to the sides as they are suctioned out. Its diameter is wide enough (.9 mm) so the eggs will not be distorted into a "sausage shape" to make their way through the opening.[5] Into the third incision, just below the navel, goes the laparoscope. Carbon dioxide gas pumped into the abdomen enhances visibility and eases access.[6]

The laparoscope, a thin instrument "about as big around as a fountain pen and twice as long," literally translates from the Greek to mean "look into the abdomen." It has a light and a lens at the end and is like a telescope or a submarine periscope. The surgeon balances the laparoscope against his or her cheek and looks for the ovaries and follicles. Until this point the follicles have only been seen as greyish, fuzzy, oval shapes on the ultrasound screen. Inside the body they stand out against the pink abdominal area and darker red ovaries. The ideal follicle looks like "a small white button mushroom, lightly criss-crossed with veins."[7] A less desirable follicle is deep blue or purple and heavily vascular.[8] Each in turn is pierced and suctioned with a foot-controlled vacuum pump.[9] A desirable place is located on the follicle that is fairly thick (so it will not tear) and without veins (so little bleeding will be induced). At that point a little pressure is exerted on the teflon-lined needle, the follicle indents, the needle is turned, and the surface is penetrated.[10]

148

The contents of the follicle are pumped out (aspirated) and the fluid goes directly into a test tube. The fluid is ideally "thin honey-coloured"[11] but by the end of the aspiration it is blood-stained. The less-than-ideal follicles yield bloody and thick fluid from the start.[12] By this time the follicle is "a collapsed sack"[13] but, after 15–20 seconds a solution is injected to fill it up again and it is aspirated a second time. The procedure may be repeated several times to ensure that no eggs are left behind, although most eggs are found in the first aspiration.[14] Aspirations are done on each follicle, which can range in number from two (the minimum desired for surgery) to eighteen or more.

It is increasingly common to replace the laparoscopy with an aspiration conducted in an office procedure with physicians watching the process through ultrasound. The suctioning needle may be inserted through the abdomen and bladder or through the vagina. The technique does not require general anesthesia, is less expensive than the laparoscopy, and may be preferable when a patient has severe adhesions that would, with a laparoscopy, have to be cleared with a preparatory surgery.[15]

The test tubes are taken to a laboratory where technicians examine the fluid for eggs. Most of the time, around 85 percent, technicians find eggs. The egg is a microscopic single-cell entity surrounded by a protective membrane of cumulus cells.[16] It is the largest of the body cells. "Illuminated from underneath," writes one author, the human egg is merely a tiny blob of jelly; a single cell buoyed up by the sticky mass in which it floated in the follicle."[17] The mass makes it barely visible to the naked eye. Each egg, as seen in a recently published book containing full-size color photographs of eggs at various stages of development,[18] has idiosyncratic traits. If the cumulus is "loosely expanded," it is a sign the egg is mature and needs to be cultured in a medium for only five or six hours. A "tightly clustered" cumulus, on the other hand, indicates an immature egg that must be cultured in a medium for twenty-four or more hours.[19] Some eggs are unfertilizable dark, solid masses—mere "greasespots."

If eggs are found in the fluid, the husband is asked to produce a semen sample. The spermatozoa in the semen also differ in quality according to number, motility, direction of movement, shape, and ability to penetrate an egg. A healthy spermatozoan swims with its head first and is oval shaped; abnormal sperm (usually making up 15 percent of the total) have heads that are too large or small, defects in the tail, or sluggish motility.[20] Because sperm lose potency with repeated ejaculations in a short period of time, the husband is asked not to ejaculate in the days preceding the expected data of laparoscopy. The spermatozoa given on that date are treated in the laboratory as the eggs mature in culture. The technician separates the sperm from the seminal fluid by spinning them so that the sperm "swim up." From 50,000 to 100,000 sperm are used for the fertilization.[21]

During fertilization, each egg is put in a glass dish and combined with some of the sperm. The egg lies on the bottom of the dish and the sperm, which are swimming, are pulled toward the egg by the force of gravity.[22] Conditions at this point are carefully monitored in light of experience that has shown any number of external events can interfere with fertilization. A glass dish is used rather than plastic, for example, because scratched plastic may release harmful substances; plastic with a nob on the bottom may also trap the eggs or sperm. The dishes are rinsed with purified water and the type of dish will have been tested beforehand, for example, by putting sperm in them to make sure they are not exuding harmful substances.[23] An embryologist with a good record of fertilizations at one center moved to another and was not achieving fertilization rates until he changed the water, suggesting that the city's water supply contained a substance that interfered with fertilization.[24]

The dishes with the eggs and sperm go into an incubator with a temperature and moisture level approximating that of the fallopian tubes. Most of the time a fertilization occurs. When one spermatozoan penetrates an egg, "a granular barrier forms which blocks the advance of other sperm."[25] The egg then undergoes a change in which a second body, the pronucleus, joins the already existing pronucleus. If two pronuclei are visible under the microscope around sixteen hours after insemination, a fertilization has occurred. If three are visible, more than one sperm has entered the egg, which leaves the egg polyspermic and unusable. If the fertilized egg were in the human body, enzymes and cilia in the fallopian tubes would remove the sticky cumulus cells. In fertilization in a glass dish, a technician removes the cumulus cells with a pipette.

Approximately eighteen hours after fertilization, the egg divides into two cells. Ideally, the cells will be of equal size, looking, as one embryologist put it, like the Olympiad logo but with only two circles. Approximately six hours later each cell divides and the egg becomes a four-celled entity. Divisions proceed in this rippling fashion as each cell divides and then each new cell divides. The embryos, technically known as preimplantation embryos, each take on their own appearances and are graded by the technicians. A good embryo has clear cells of relatively equal size and shape that each have one nucleus. The cells of a poor embryo have several nuclei, are of unequal size and uneven shape, and are fragmented.[26] In nature, up to two-thirds of embryos are silently sloughed from the body and many of these are thought to be of poor quality. One of the recurring questions of IVF is whether to use poor quality embryos. Generally most embryos are transferred, irrespective of their appearance because the science of knowing whether appearance makes a difference is imperfect and it is assumed the body will slough the abnormal ones in any case.

Most IVF centers transfer the embryos to the woman's uterus when the embryos are at the four- or eight-cell stage. The embryo transfer itself is a simple procedure, performed in an office. The woman lies on a table, either on her back with head slightly lower than her feet or facing down with her knees to her chest, depending on the tilt of her uterus. In the adjoining laboratory, the embryologist loads the embryos, with a small amount of culture medium, into a catheter. The physician then inserts the catheter into the vagina and through the cervix. The embryos are released. If the transfer is being monitored by ultrasound, the release of fluid is visible on the screen. The catheter is then examined under the microscope to make sure no embryos remain.[27]

The woman rests in a recovery room for six to eight hours and then leaves the hospital for two to three days of bedrest. Two weeks later, if menstruation has not started, her blood is tested to detect the chemical changes associated with pregnancy. It is not unusual for a blood draw to make it appear the woman is pregnant when in fact she is not. This is known as a chemical pregnancy. A true (clinical) pregnancy is determined by the visibility of a fetus on ultrasound twelve weeks after transfer.

Scientifically speaking, IVF is simple and holds promises for more streamlining. Already, the techniques of early IVF seem primitive. Within ten years, vaginal extraction of ova, improvements in endocrinology, the ability to microinject eggs with sperm, and the freezing of eggs and embryos will be among the techniques that make up IVF.

Notes

1. BEGINNING AN ERA OF CHOICE

1. "Invit: The View from the Glass Oviduct," *Saturday Review*, September 30, 1972, p. 68.
2. Michael S. Gregory, "Science and Humanities: Toward A New World View," in D. Heyward Brock, ed., *The Culture of Biomedicine: Studies in Science and Culture*, 1:21.
3. Quoted in *ibid.*, pp. 21–22.
4. Lisa Belkin, "Consumers Confused by Number of Choices," *New York Times*, August 8, 1985, p. 1.
5. Elizabeth Neuffer, "Galaxy of Microwave Foods Is Expanding," *New York Times*, February 17, 1988, p. D1.

2. TRACKING THE SYMBOLS OF IN VITRO FERTILIZATION

1. Alfred North Whitehead, *Symbolism: Its Meaning and Effect*, p. 6.
2. "Test-Tube Babies Pilloried Again," *Nature*, February 4, 1982, 295:445.
3. Alan F. Guttmacher, "Early Attitudes Toward Infertility," pp. 9 and 7.
4. Harold Speert, "Historical Introduction," in Landrum B. Shettles, *Ovum Humanum*, p. vii.
5. Gena Corea, *The Mother Machine: Reproductive Technologies from Artificial Insemination to Artificial Wombs*, pp. 326–327.
6. See sources listed in Landrum B. Shettles, "A Morula Stage of Human Ovum Developed In Vitro."

7. Speert, "Historical Introduction," p. viii.
8. R. G. Edwards, B. D. Bavister, and P. C. Steptoe, "Early Stages of Fertilization *In Vitro* of Human Ooctyes," *Nature*, February 15, 1969, 221:632–635.
9. Robert G. Edwards and Patrick Steptoe, *A Matter of Life*, pp. 89–90, 94.
10. *Ibid.*, pp. 66, 47, and 101.
11. Amitai Etzioni, *Genetic Fix*, p. 59.
12. Aldous Huxley, *Brave New World*.
13. *New York Times* quoted in Edwards and Steptoe, *Matter of Life*, p. 83; D. M. Rorvik, "The Test-Tube Baby Is Coming," *Look*, May 18, 1971, p. 83.
14. Bruce Hilton, "The Seeds of Doubt," *The Record*, March 26, 1972.
15. Quoted in Edwards and Steptoe, *Matter of Life*, p. 84.
16. Leon R. Kass, "Making Babies—The New Biology and the 'Old' Mortality," *Public Interest* (Winter 1972), 26:18–56; and Paul Ramsey, "Shall We 'Reproduce'?"
17. See, for example, Joseph Fletcher in Gebhard F. B. Schumacher et al., "In Vitro Fertilization of Human Ova and Blastocyst Transfer: An Invitational Symposium."
18. Leon R. Kass, "Babies by Means of In Vitro Fertilization: Unethical Experiments on the Unborn?" *New England Journal of Medicine* (1971), 285:1174–1179; James D. Watson, "Moving Toward the Clonal Man—Is This What We Want? *Congressional Record*, U.S. Senate, April 29, 1971, pp. 12751–12752; and, Ramsey, "Reproduce?"
19. P. C. Steptoe, R. G. Edwards, and G. M. Purdy, "Human Blastocysts Grown in Culture," *Nature* (1971), 229:132–133; R. G. Edwards et al., "Factors Influencing the Success of In Vitro Fertilization for Alleviating Human Infertility."
20. Ronald A. Carson, "Paul Ramsey, Principled Protestant Casuist: A Retrospective," *Medical Humanities Review* (January 1988), 2:26.
21. Edwards and Steptoe, *Matter of Life*, p. 113.
22. Ramsy, "Reproduce?" p. 1481.
23. Judith Cummings, "Gynecologist's Letter Challenges Couple in 'Test-Tube Baby' Case," *New York Times*, July 22, 1978, p. 24; and "Childless Couple Is Suing Doctor," *New York Times*, July 16, 1978, p. 26.
24. Transcript of tape-recorded conversation between Drs. Raymond Vande Wiele, Landrum Shettles, and W. Duane Todd, pp. 9–10.
25. Judith Cummings, "Doctor Says She Alerted Chief on 'Test-Tube' Baby," *New York Times*, August 5, 1978, p. 23.
26. The conversation was recorded secretly by Vande Wiele and was introduced as evidence in the trial.
27. This was an incorrect supposition. An official at the National Institutes of Health said the NIH had not banned IVF experimentation. Judith Cummings, "U.S. Aide Denies Ban on Embryo Testing," *New York Times*, July 20, 1978, p. B13.

28. The transcript showed Vande Wiele was angry about published comments by Shettles to the effect that there were no ethical problems with IVF. "Transcript," pp. 6–8.

29. Judith Cummings, "Doctor Defends His Procedures in 'Test-Tube Baby' Experiment," *New York Times*, July 21, 1978, p. A14.

30. Peter Singer and Deane Wells, *The Reproductive Revolution*, p. 48. They asked for $1.5 million.

31. Sharon Churcher, " 'Test-Tube Mom Was Pawn in Doctor's Quest for Glory,' " *New York Post*, July 18, 1978, p. 3, quoting the hospital lawyer.

32. Cummings, "Doctor Defends," quoting Doris Del Zio's physician.

33. P. C. Steptoe and R. G. Edwards, "Birth After the Reimplantation of a Human Embryo," *Lancet* (1978), 2:683.

34. *New York Daily News*, July 29, 1978.

35. *New York Times*, July 27, 1978, p. A16.

36. British headline photographed and reprinted in *ibid.*

37. *People*, March 5, 1984, p. 73. See Sherman Elias and George J. Annas, "Social Policy Considerations in Noncoital Reproduction," p. 62. She was chosen "by simply being."

38. Quoted in Edwards and Steptoe, *Matter of Life*, p. 84.

39. Ethics Advisory Board, Department of Health, Education, and Welfare, *Appendix: HEW Support of Research Involving Human IN VITRO Fertilization and Embryo Transfer*. See also "This Is What You Thought About . . . Test-Tube Babies," *Glamour*, June 1982, 80:29.

40. "Doctor Doubts Ethics in Case of British Baby," *New York Times*, July 27, 1978, p. A16.

41. "Childless Couple Is Suing Doctor," *New York Times*, July 16, 1978, p. 26.

42. National Council of the Society for the Protection of Unborn Children, "Man's Intrusion on Nature," in Jerome Lejeune and Paul Ramsey, *The Question of In Vitro Fertilization: Studies in Medicine, Law and Ethics*, p. 55. In England, gynecologists who refused to do abortions were sent to infertility clinics to compensate (pp. 55–56).

43. Virginia L. Warren, "A Powerful Metaphor: Medicine Is War," unpublished paper.

44. Paul Hodgkin, "Medicine Is War: And Other Medical Metaphors," p. 1820.

45. National Council, "Man's Intrusion," p. 69. See also Leon R. Kass, *Toward a More Natural Science*, pp. 121–123.

46. Harriet F. Simons, "Infertility: Implications for Policy Formulation," in Miriam D. Mazor and Harriet F. Simons, *Infertility: Medical, Emotional and Social Considerations*, p. 64.

47. Quoted in Walter Wadlington, "Artificial Conception: The Challenge for Family Law," p. 465.

48. Quoted in Simons, "Infertility," p. 64.

49. Hans O. Tiefel, "Human In Vitro Fertilization: A Conservative View," p. 3238.

50. Simons, "Infertility," p. 65.

51. Quoted in Guttmacher, "Early Attitudes," p. 4.

52. *Ibid.*, p. 3, referring to the 811 prescriptions found on ancient Egyptian papyri.

53. G. L. Christie, "The Psychological and Social Management of the Infertile Couple," p. 238.

54. Albert Decker and Suzanne Loebl, *Why Can't We Have a Baby?* p. 36.

55. See Christie, "Psychological Management," pp. 233–237, for a summary of some of these theories.

56. Described in Christie. For citations of other studies, see C. H. Garner, "Psychological Aspects of IVF and the Infertile Couple," in Christopher M. Fredericks et al., eds., *Foundations of In Vitro Fertilization,* pp. 305–306.

57. Miriam D. Mazor, "Emotional Reactions to Infertility," in Mazor and Simons, *Infertility,* pp. 23–24.

58. Decker and Loebl, *Why Can't We?* p. 35.

59. *Doornbos v. Doornbos,* No. 54 S. 1498 (Superior Court, Cook Co., December 13, 1954).

60. R. J. Aitken and D. W. Lincoln, "Human Embryo Research: The Case for Contraception," in CIBA Foundation, *Human Embryo Research: Yes or No?* pp. 122–136.

61. Edwards and Steptoe, *Matter of Life,* pp. 73–75.

62. Barbara Eck Menning, *Infertility: A Guide for the Childless Couple.*

63. Diane Clapp, "Emotional Responses to Infertility."

64. Garner, "Psychological Aspects," p. 306.

65. *Roe v. Wade,* 410 U. S. 113 (1973).

66. OTA Report Brief, "Infertility: Medical and Social Choices." See also Sevgi O. Aral, et al., "The Increasing Concern With Infertility."

67. "What You Should Know About Infertility," *Contemporary OB/GYN* (February 1980), 101:101; Clifford Grobstein et al., "External Human Fertilization: An Evaluation of Policy."

68. Jaroslav F. Hulka, "Diagnosis and Treatment of Tubal Disease," in Mary G. Hammond and Luther M. Talbert, eds., *Infertility: Practical Guide for the Physician,* p. 114, footnote omitted.

69. Lori B. Andrews, *New Conceptions: A Consumer's Guide to the Newest Infertility Treatments,* p. 27.

70. Grobstein, et al., "External Human Fertilization," p. 130.

71. Ethics Advisory Board, Department of Health, Education, and Welfare, *Report and Conclusions: HEW Support of Research Involving Human In Vitro Fertilization and Embryo Transfer,* p. 38.

72. Janice Perry, "Researchers Set Sights on Cure for Infertility," *Chicago Tribune,* November 11, 1984, p. 3, sec. 6.

73. Jouke Halme, "In Vitro Fertilization—A New Treatment for Infertility," in Hammond and Talbert, *Infertility*, p. 181.

74. Wadlington, "Artificial Conception," p. 466. See also Robert Lindsey, "Adoption Market: Big Demand, Tight Supply," *New York Times*, April 5, 1987, p. 1.

75. Lawyer quoted in Alan L. Otten, "Medical Efforts to Help Childless Couples Pose Host of Difficult Issues," *Wall Street Journal*, August 7, 1984, p. 13.

76. Gina Kolata, "In Vitro Fertilization Goes Commercial," *Science*, September 16, 1983, 221:1160.

77. Halme, "In Vitro Fertilization," p. 187.

78. Whitehead, *Symbolism*, p. 61.

3. THE RESPONSIBLE PHYSICIAN

1. Gary B. Ellis, Office of Technology Assessment. Presentation at University of Virginia Reproductive Sciences Seminar Series, May 6, 1988.

2. Sandra Blakeslee, "Trying to Make Money Making 'Test-Tube' Babies," *New York Times*, May 17, 1987, p. 6, sec. 6.

3. Machelle M. Seibel, "A New Era in Reproductive Technology"; and Blakeslee, "Trying to Make Money."

4. Blakeslee, "Trying to Make Money."

5. For example, the eyes of Georgeanna Jones, a pioneer of IVF technology in this country, reportedly filled with tears when she was criticized by right-to-life groups because she was thinking about the "women she was treating." Deborah Marquardt, "Georgeanna Jones," *Commonwealth* (September 1982), p. 74.

6. R. G. Edwards and Patrick Steptoe, *A Matter of Life*, p. 39.

7. *Ibid.*, p. 109; and *Hearings on Human Embryo Transfer*, p. 41 (testimony of Howard W. Jones, Jr.).

8. Sharon Churcher, in *New York Post*, July 18, 1978, p. 3.

9. The conditions of IVF may play a role in low embryo implantation rates. See, for example, Maria F. Hayes et al., "Effect of General Anesthesia on Fertilization and Cleavage of Human Oocytes In Vitro."

10. On the number of embryos transferred at a time, see R. G. Edwards and P. C. Steptoe, "Current Status of In-Vitro Fertilisation and Implantation of Human Embryos," *Lancet* (December 3, 1983), 8362:1265–1269; Esther Eisenberg and Edward E. Wallach, "In Vitro Fertilization and Embryo Transfer," *Postgraduate Obstetrics and Gynecology* (September 1984), 4:1–5.

11. Andrea L. Bonnicksen and Robert H. Blank, "The Government and In Vitro Fertilization (IVF): Views of IVF Directors."

12. Medical Research International, American Fertility Society Special Inter-

est Group, "In Vitro Fertilization/ Embryo Transfer in the United States: 1985 and 1986 Results from the National IVF/ET Registry."

13. Seibel, "New Era."

14. Unpublished results of survey of IVF directors conducted in the spring of 1987. See Bonnicksen and Blank, "The Government and IVF."

15. "Ethical Statement on In Vitro Fertilization," *Fertility and Sterility* (January 1984), 41:13; Ethics Committee of the American Fertility Society, "Ethical Considerations of the New Reproductive Technologies."

16. "Ethical Statement."

17. David T. Ozar, "The Case Against Thawing Unused Frozen Embryos."

18. Lori B. Andrews, "Legal and Ethical Aspects of New Reproductive Technologies."

19. See scientific articles cited in Andrea L. Bonnicksen, "Advocacy of Human Embryo Research: Emerging Values."

20. For a discussion of the gatekeeping role of physicians, see Eugene B. Brody, "Reproduction Without Sex—But with the Doctor."

21. Roslyn R. Angell, A. A. Templeton, and R. J. Aitken, "Chromosomal Studies in Human In Vitro Fertilization."

22. J. L. Watt et al., "Trisomy 1 in an Eight Cell Human Pre-Embryo."

23. Sally Engle Merry, "Concepts of Law and Justice Among Working-Class Americans: Ideology as Culture."

24. Maria Bustillo et al., "Delivery of a Healthy Infant Following Nonsurgical Ovum Transfer."

25. "Human Embryo Research: Vote for Progress." In Britain, more openness about embryo research occurs as a result of oversight by the Voluntary Licensing Authority. See VLA Secretariat, "The Third Report of the Voluntary Licensing Authority for Human *In Vitro* Fertilisation and Embryology."

26. John A. Robertson, "Embryos, Families, and Procreative Liberty: The Legal Structure of the New Reproduction."

27. CIBA Foundation, *Human Embryo Research: Yes or No?* p. 116.

28. D. J. Weatherall et al., "Analysis of Foetal DNA for the Diagnosis and Management of Genetic Disease," in CIBA Foundation, *Human Embryo Research*, pp. 83–100.

29. Reprinted in Tom L. Beauchamp and James F. Childress, *Principles of Biomedical Ethics*, pp. 329–330.

30. Leon R. Kass, "Ethical Dilemmas in the Care of the Ill, Part I. What Is the Physician's Service?" p. 1816.

31. *Ibid.*

32. Leon R. Kass, "Ethical Dilemmas in the Care of the Ill, Part II. What Is the Patient's Good?" p. 1946.

33. C. H. Garner, "Psychological Aspects of IVF and the Infertile Couple," in Christopher M. Fredericks et al., eds. p. 309.

34. Kass, "Ethical Dilemmas, Part II," p. 1949.

35. See, for example, Edmund D. Pellegrino, "The Anatomy of Clinical-

4. The Responsible Patient

Ethical Judgments in Perinatology and Neonatology: A Substantive and Procedural Framework."
36. *Ibid.*, p. 209.
37. Edwards and Steptoe, *Matter of Life*, p. 39.
38. "French Researcher Says 'Non' to Egg Manipulation."
39. Kass, "Ethical Dilemmas, Part I," p. 1815.
40. "Baby Craving," *Life* (June 1987), pp. 36–42.
41. Edwards and Steptoe, *Matter of Life*, p. 59.
42. *Ibid.*, p. 79. For other examples of early research involving women about to undergo hysterectomies, done with their consent, see Gebhard F. B. Schumacher et al., "In Vitro Fertilization of Human Ova and Blastocyst Transfer," p. 195.

4. THE RESPONSIBLE PATIENT

1. Edmund D. Pellegrino, *Humanism and the Physician*, p. 225.
2. Quoted in Gena Corea, *The Mother Machine; Reproductive Technologies from Artificial Insemination to Artificial Wombs*, p. 167. The mother of another early IVF baby said, "I never asked if they had any successes. I was too polite to ask that question" (p. 168).
3. Marge Brown, "Having It All," *Resolve Newsletter*, September 1987, p. 71.
4. Barbara Eck Menning, *Infertility: A Guide for the Childless Couple*, p. 126.
5. Cynthia Laitman Orenberg, *DES: The Complete Story* (New York: St. Martin's Press, 1981), p. 56. The word derives from hystero (uterus), salpingo (tube), gamma (written). Albert Decker and Suzanne Loebl, *Why Can't We Have a Baby?"* p. 86.
6. Eck Menning, *Infertility*, pp. 96–102.
7. *Ibid.*, p. 110, quoting an infertile woman.
8. *Ibid.*, p. 110.
9. Phyllis C. Leppert and Barbara S. Pahlka, "Grieving Characteristics After Spontaneous Abortion: A Management Approach," *Obstetrics and Gynecology* (July 1984), 64:121.
10. Ronni Batterman, "A Comprehensive Approach to Treating Infertility," p. 47.
11. Linda Salzer, counselor for Resolve, speaking at the Hastings Center, Briarcliff Manor, N.Y., September 23, 1987.
12. Quoted in Lori B. Andrews, *New Conceptions: A Consumer's Guide to the Newest Infertility Treatment*, p. 97.
13. Ellen W. Freeman et al., "Psychological Evaluation and Support in a Program of In Vitro Fertilization and Embryo Transfer," p. 50.
14. Salzer, remarks.
15. Eck Menning, *Infertility*, pp. 68–69.
16. Batterman, "Comprehensive Approach."

159

17. Tom L. Beauchamp and James F. Childress, *Principles of Biomedical Ethics*, pp. 168–182.

18. Edmund D. Pellegrino, "Anatomy of Clinical-Ethical Judgments in Perinatology and Neonatology," p. 204.

19. Quoted in Harriet F. Simons, "Infertility: Implications for Policy Formulation," in Mazor and Simons, *Infertility*, p. 63.

20. Cheryl F. McCartney, "The Doctor-Patient Relationship in Infertility Therapy," in Mary G. Hammond and Luther M. Talbert, eds., *Infertility: Practical Guide for the Physician*, p. 18.

21. Freeman et al., "Psychological Evaluation," p. 51.

22. Data from one hospital reporting in 1988. See Machelle M. Seibel, "A New Era in Reproductive Technology," p. 829.

23. *Ibid.*, p. 831.

24. *Ibid.*

25. Medical Research International, "IVF/ET."

26. Batterman, "Comprehensive Approach," p. 48.

27. Peter Roberts, "The Brennan Story: A Small Miracle of Creation," in William A. W. Walters and Peter Singer, eds., *Test-Tube Babies: A Guide to Moral Questions, Present Techniques and Future Possibilities*, p. 13.

28. Pellegrino, "Anatomy," p. 204.

29. Boston Women's Health Book Collective, *Our Bodies, Ourselves*, 2d ed. (New York: Simon and Schuster, 1976).

30. Jeff and Karen Stewart, "How to Stand in Line for a Miracle." Letter posted at the Center for Fertility and Reproductive Research, Vanderbilt University Medical Center.

31. Freeman et al., "Psychological Evaluation"; C. H. Garner, "Psychological Aspects of IVF and the Infertile Couple," in Christopher M. Fredericks et al., *Foundations of In Vitro Fertilization;* Patricia Mahlstedt and Linda R. Applegarth, "The Psychosocial Issues of In Virto Fertilization: Coping and Control" pp. 83–86.

32. McCartney, "Doctor-Patient," p. 23.

33. Isabel Bainbridge, "With Child in Mind: The Experience of a Potential IVF Mother," in William A. W. Walters and Peter Singer eds., *Test-Tube Babies: A Guide to Moral Questions, Present Techniques and Future Possibilities*, p. 124.

34. Sandra Blakeslee, "Trying to Make Money Making 'Test-Tube' Babies."

35. Michael R. Soules, "The In Vitro Fertilization Pregnancy Rate: Let's Be Honest with One Another," *Fertility and Sterility* (April 1985), 43:511–513.

36. R. G. Edwards and Patrick C. Steptoe, "Current Status of In Vitro Fertilisation and Implantation of Human Embryos," *Lancet* (Dec. 3, 1983), 8362:1265–1269; Esther Eisenberg and Edward E. Wallach, "In Vitro Fertilization and Embryo Transfer," *Postgraduate Obstetrics and Gynecology* (Sept. 1984), 4:1–5.

37. National Perinatal Statistics Unit, *In Vitro Fertilization Pregnancies—Australia 1980–1893*, p. 15.

38. Alberto Romeu et al., "Results of In Vitro Fertilization Attempts in Women 40 Years of Age and Older: The Norfolk Experience"; and C. Campagnoli et al., "Patient Selection for In Vitro Fertilization (IVF) and Embryo Transfer (ET)."

39. National Perinatal Unit, *Pregnancies 1980–1983*, p. 12.

40. Rodney Lyles et al., "Characterization and Response of Women Undergoing Repeat Cycles of Ovulation Induction in an In Vitro Fertilization and Embryo Transfer Program."

41. Campagnoli, "Patient Selection," p. 1492; and Claudio F. Chillik, "The Role of In Vitro Fertilization in Infertile Patients with Endometriosis." This was not for mild or moderate endometriosis.

42. For an example of a study in which the authors concluded it was effective, see G. R. Hull et al., "Population Study of Causes, Treatment, and Outcome of Infertility," pp. 1693–1697.

43. Perri Klass, *A Not Entirely Benign Procedure: Four Years as a Medical Student* (New York: Putnam, 1987), p. 50.

5. A RESPONSIBLE GOVERNMENT

1. Morris B. Abram and Susan M. Wolf, "Public Involvement in Medical Ethics," p. 629.

2. See, for example, *Griswold v. Connecticut*, 381 U.S. 479 (1965); *Eisenstadt v. Baird*, 405 U.S. 438 (1972).

3. Kathryn Venturatos-Lorio, "Alternative Means of Reproduction: Virgin Territory for Legislation"; p. 1676; Harry D. Krause, "Artificial Conception: Legislative Approaches," p. 190; *Hearings on Embryo Transfer*, pp. 344, 346.

4. Soupart gave permission for the proposal to be made public in a letter to the Secretary of the Department of Health, Education, and Welfare on August 15, 1978. The proposal is hereinafter cited as "Soupart Proposal."

5. James D. Watson, "Moving Toward the Clonal Man," in the *Congressional Record;* Watson, "Moving Toward the Clonal Man: Is This What We Want?" *Atlantic Monthly*, May 1971, 227:50–53; Alvin Toffler, *Future Shock* (New York: Random House, 1970); and Amitai Etzioni, *Genetic Fix*, p. 16.

6. *Roe v. Wade*, 410 U. S. 113 (1973).

7. Lori B. Andrews, "Legal and Ethical Aspects of New Reproductive Technologies," p. 194.

8. For a history of the drafts of the final policy, see Ethics Advisory Board, *Report and Conclusions*.

9. *Federal Register* 40:33527 (August 8, 1975); 45 C.F.R. s. 46.204(d).

10. He planned to use a maximum of three patients per week for forty-five weeks of the year for three years. He would tell the women they would gain "no benefit" from participation in the study. "Soupart Proposal," pp. 49, 54. He

hoped to fertilize around 450 eggs. Leon R. Kass, *Toward a More Natural Science*, p. 100.

11. Kass, *Natural Science*, p. 100.

12. "Soupart Proposal," p. 36.

13. EAB, *Report and Conclusions*, reprinted in Clifford Grobstein, *From Chance to Purpose*, pp. 159–204.

14. "Memorandum for the Honorable James C. Gaither, Chairman, the Ethics Advisory Board of HEW," from Joseph A. Califano, Jr., September 15, 1978, reprinted in Grobstein, *Chance to Purpose*, pp. 155–156.

15. Bethesda, Boston, Seattle, San Francisco, Atlanta, Kansas City, Detroit, Philadelphia, Denver, Dallas, and New York City. EAB Report and Conclusions, reprinted in Grobstein, *Chance to Purpose*, p. 194.

16. EAB, *Appendix: HEW Support*.

17. *Federal Register* 35033-35058 (June 18, 1979).

18. Krause, "Artificial Conception," p. 190, described it as "thoughtful."

19. The Board did not elaborate on the reason for selecting fourteen days as a limit other than to note that fourteen days was the stage "normally associated with the completion of implantation." EAB, *Report and Conclusions*, reprinted in Grobstein, *Chance to Purpose*, p. 201.

20. The Board identified the National Institute of Child Health and Human Development in particular as an agency that could work with others to help collect information from IVF practitioners here and abroad and develop a systematic way of collecting that information.

21. Clifford Grobstein concluded that "one cannot help but remark that the Commission recognized a hot potato when it saw one." Grobstein, *Chance to Purpose*, p. 114.

22. John Mendeloff, "Politics and Bioethical Commissions: 'Muddling Through' and the 'Slippery Slope,' " p. 87.

23. Most came from the Midwest, New York, and New Jersey. Office for Protection from Research Risks, Office of the Director, National Institutes of Health, "Report on The Public Response to *In Vitro* Fertilization and Embryo Transfer," April 15, 1980, pp. 5, i, 3. The organization sending 25,000 signed petitions was not named in the report.

24. *Ibid.*, pp. i–ii.

25. *Ibid.*, p. v.

26. The writer of this letter thought that infertile couples were suffering during the time it was taking the Department of Health, Education, and Welfare to reach a decision. *Ibid.*, p. v.

27. The commission, called the Commission for the Study of Ethical Problems in Medicine and Biomedical and Behavioral Research, took the place of the National Commission for the Protection of Human Subjects. Grobstein, *Chance to Purpose*, p. 138. Senators Orin Hatch and Edward Kennedy asked for the review on February 21, 1980. Grobstein, *Chance to Purpose*, p. 114.

28. Barbara Mishkin, quoted in Philip M. Boffey, "Doctrine Follows Years of Debate on Procedures," *New York Times*, March 12, 1987, p. 13.

29. No letter is on the record at the Department of Health and Human Services (formerly Department of Health, Education, and Welfare). For a comment on the disbanding, see *Hearings on Embryo Transfer* (testimony of Samuel Gorovitz), p. 368.

30. "Genetic Engineering in Man: Ethical Considerations," Editorial, *Journal of the American Medical Association* (May 1, 1972), 220:721.

31. Barbara Mishkin, quoted in Boffey, "Doctrine Follows Debate."

32. Califano's job loss as Secretary of DHEW, which occurred shortly after he received the EAB report, may have been related in part to the report. *Hearings on Embryo Transfer*, p. 368.

33. Alan L. Otten, "Infertility Enterprises Give Birth to Concern."

34. Gina Kolata, "Ethics and Fetal Research: Government Begins to Move," *New York Times*, July 31, 1988, p. E7; Warren E. Leary, "Panel to Back Fertility Study Is Revived," *New York Times*, July 15, 1988, p. 6; *Federal Register*, September 12, 1988, pp. 35232–35233.

36. See, for example, the prepared statements of Gary B. Ellis and Richard P. Marrs in *Hearings on Consumer Protection Issues Involving In Vitro Fertilization Clinics;* and the prepared statement of George J. Annas in *Hearings on Alternative Reproductive Technologies: Implications for Children and Families*, pp. 102–114.

37. "Minimal Standards for Programs of In Vitro Fertilization," *Fertility and Sterility* (January 1984) 41:13.

38. Krause, "Artificial Conception," p. 198. But see Lori Andrews, testifying in *Hearings on Embryo Transfer*, p. 164, who noted that by and large, "traditional mechanisms" of regulation, such as large malpractice suits "do not operate as forcefully with respect to the new reproductive technologies" as in other areas of medicine." On questions of liability and IVF, see I. R. Hill, "Liability and In-Vitro Fertilization."

39. *In re Baby M*, 13 F.L.R. 2001, April 7, 1987.

40. Ivar Peterson, "States Assess Surrogate Motherhood," *New York Times*, December 13, 1987, p. 42.

41. See, for example, the prepared statement of Carol Peters in *Hearings on Consumer Protection Issues.*

42. Medical Research International, "IVF/ET," p. 214.

43. National Perinatal Statistics Unit, Fertility Society of Australia. *In Vitro Fertilisation Pregnancies, Australia and New Zealand, 1979–1986.* Sydney: NPSU, 1987.

44. See, for example, B. Bourrit et al., "Psychotic Reaction After in Vitro Fertilization (IVF)," Letter to Editor, *Journal of In Vitro Fertilization and Embryo Transfer* (April 1988) 5:114.

45. Ethics Committee, AFS, "Ethical Considerations," pp. 90S–94S; prepared statement of Richard P. Marrs in *Hearings on Consumer Protection Issues.*

Other groups within the AFS include the Society of Reproductive Endocrinologists and the Society of Reparative Surgeons.

46. Medical Research International, "IVF/ET."

47. Machelle E. Seibel, "A New Era in Reproductive Technology," p. 834.

48. Committee on Ethics, American College of Obstetricians and Gynecologists, "ACOG Committee Statement: Ethical Issues in Human In Vitro Fertilization and Embryo Placement," 1986, p. 3 (referring to last quote only).

49. *Hearings on Embryo Transfer* (testimony of Howard W. Jones, Jr.), p. 43. The AFS committee recommended personnel requirements and other services that ought to be available such as 24-hour ultrasonography facilities. "Minimal Standards." See also Committee on Gynecologic Practice, American College of Obstetricians and Gynecologists, "ACOG Committee Statement: "Human In Vitro Fertilization and Embryo Placement," 1984.

50. In Ethics Committee, AFS, "Ethical Considerations," for example, Richard McCormick, a Catholic theologian, approved the principle of IVF research and practice. See Rev. Richard A. McCormick, "Ethics of Reproductive Technology: AFS Recommendations, Dissent."

51. Committee on Ethics, "ACOG Committee Statement," p. 3.

52. Press release of the American Fertility Society, March 1987.

53. Ethics Committee, AFS, "Ethical Considerations," pp. 46S, 18S, 61S.

54. *Ibid.*, pp. 56S–57S, suggested that research would lead to knowledge to help identify abnormalities in embryos.

55. The committee referred to the "production" and "generation" of embryos but did not make clear whether this meant the creation of embryos for research purposes through such techniques as twinning. *Ibid.*, p. 57S.

56. *Ibid.*, pp. 56S, and 3S–4S.

57. *Ibid.*, p. 57S. The final statement reiterated that the government should be encouraged to fund "innovative reproductive research proposals" (p. 78S).

58. Howard W. Jones, Jr., quoted in Joel Brinkley, "Uncertain Present for In Vitro Fertilization," *New York Times*, February 5, 1984, p. 20E.

59. Ethics Committee, AFS, "Ethical Considerations," pp. 77S–78S.

60. "The married couple's right to reproduce should thus extend to noncoital means of conception, which include the wide range of choices made possible by developments in IVF." *Ibid.*, p. 4S.

61. "The donors therefore have the right to decide at their sole discretion the disposition of these items [gametes and concepti], provided such disposition is within medical and ethical guidelines as outlined herein." "Ethical Statement" (1984).

62. For a contractual approach to the use of tissues, see Ethics Committee, AFS, "Ethical Considerations," p. 4S. See also *Hearings on Embryo Transfer*, p. 68, for this exchange between subcommittee chair Albert Gore, Jr., and Howard W. Jones, Jr. about the 1984 AFS "Ethical Statement":

Gore: "Would you also say that the embryos are the property of the donors?"

Jones: "Well, I think the word property here is used in the sense of the parents having a certain say in the ultimate disposition of them."

63. *Hearings on Embryo Transfer*, pp. 1–2.

64. *Ibid.*, pp. 344 (testimony of S. Gorovitz) and 218 (testimony of George J. Annas).

65. Mary Warnock, *A Question of Life: The Warnock Report on Human Fertilisation and Embryology*, p. 2.

66. Henry J. Abraham, *Freedom and the Court*, 2d ed. (New York: Oxford University Press, 1972), p. 177. From Chief Justice Warren's dissent in *Times Film Corp. v. Chicago*, 365 U.S. 43 (1961).

67. The law states that "a person shall not carry out a prohibited procedure." Elsewhere it states that "a 'prohibited procedure' means — (a) cloning." Infertility Medical Procedures Act (Vic.) 1984, s. 6(1)(2). See Margaret Brumby and Pascal Kasimba, "When Is Cloning Lawful?" p. 198.

68. Peter Singer, "Australian Developments in Reproductive Technology."

69. John A. Robertson, "The Scientist's Right to Research: A Constitutional Analysis."

70. "Where trans-species fertilisation is used . . . in the assessment or diagnosis of subfertility it should be subject to licence . . . and the development of any resultant hybrid should be terminated at the two-cell stage." Warnock, *Question of Life*, p. 71.

71. See, for example, *Schenck v. United States*, 249 U.S. 47 (1919).

72. VLA Secretariat, "The Second Report of the Voluntary Licensing Authority for Human *In Vitro* Fertilisation and Embryology," p. 1.

73. *Ibid.*, p. 11.

74. "Draft Legislation on Infertility Services and Embryo Research," *Lancet* (December 5, 1987), 2:8571:1343.

75. "Embryo Centre Fails Licensing Test," *New Scientist*, April 24, 1986, 110:24.

76. "A Once and Future Biomedical Ethics Board," *Hastings Center Report* (April/May 1988), 18:2–3.

77. Senate Bills 268 and 269 (1988). A list of these and other bills was provided by Gary B. Ellis of the Office of Technology Assessment.

78. See *Hearings on Alternative Reproductive Technologies; Hearings on Consumer Protection Issues.*

79. Prepared statement of Gary B. Ellis in *Hearings on Consumer Protection Issues*, p. 10.

80. Ira Sharkansky, *The Maligned States: Policy Accomplishments, Problems, and Opportunities*, 2d ed. (New York: McGraw-Hill, 1978), p. 2.

81. Andrea Bonnicksen and Edward Brazil, "The Policy of Alternative Conception: Looking to the States," paper presented at the 1985 American Political Science Association Annual Meeting, New Orleans, pp. 2–4.

82. *Ibid.* See Jack L. Walker, "The Diffusion of Innovations Among the American States," *American Political Science Review* (1969), 58:880–899.

83. National Conference of Commissioners on Uniform State Laws, "Status of Children of the New Biology," draft report, 1987.

84. Lori B. Andrews, "The Stork Market: The Law of the New Reproductive Technologies," p. 52.

85. Louisiana Revised Statutes, Ch. 8, 1:55.121–133. See also Office of Technology Assessment, U.S. Congress, *Infertility: Medical and Social Choices,* OTA-BA-358 (Washington, D.C.: GPO, May 1988), p. 252.

86. Bonnicksen and Brazil, "Alternative Conception," p. 4.

87. Robert Hanley, "Legislators Are Hesitant on Regulating Surrogacy," *New York Times,* February 4, 1988, p. B7.

88. *Hearings on Embryo Transfer,* p. 163 (testimony of Lori B. Andrews).

89. *Illinois Revised Statutes,* ch. 38 s. 81–26 (1983).

90. Representative Greiman recounting the question and answer in a debate in the Illinois Assembly on May 27, 1983. State of Illinois, 83rd General Assembly, House of Representatives, Transcription Debate, HB 671, p. 147.

91. Bonnicksen and Brazil, "Alternative Conception," p. 5.

92. Representative Greiman, Transcription Debate, p. 148; and Andrews, "Legal and Ethical Aspects," p. 195.

93. Andrews, *New Conceptions,* pp. 148–149.

94. On the relation between the Uniform Commercial Code and embryo trafficking, see George J. Annas, "Redefining Parenthood and Protecting Embryos: Why We Need New Laws."

95. See prepared statement of Richard P. Marrs in *Hearings on Consumer Protection Issues,* p. 6.

96. William Handel, quoted in Alan L. Otten, "Infertility Enterprises Give Birth to Concern."

97. Medical Research International, "IVF/ET."

98. Office of Technology Assessment, *Infertility: Medical and Social Choices,* p. 252.

99. Prepared statement of Richard P. Marrs in *Hearings on Consumer Protection Issues,* p. 8.

100. See, for example, George T. Sulzner, "The Policy Process and the Uses of National Governmental Study Commissions."

101. Normal Quist, "Institutional Review Boards and Human Subjects Research," p. 826.

102. Ch. 237, Laws of Maryland (1985); Ch. 5 (477E) (1986).

103. Office of Technology Assessment, *Infertility: Medical and Social Choices,* p. 150.

104. See *ibid.,* pp. 150–151, for a description of state insurance laws relating to IVF.

105. House Bills 2220, 2221, 2852, and Senate Bill 9. A list of these bills was provided by Gary B. Ellis of the Office of Technology Assessment.

106. Letter from Frank H. Murkowski to the Director of the Office of Technology Assessment, September 13, 1985

107. Representative Schroeder stated that the purpose of the bill (H.R. 2852) was to open infertility care to moderate income groups. "Who Should Pay for Infertility?", p. 4.

108. Ellen W. Freeman et al., "Psychological Evaluation and Support in a Program of In Vitro Fertilization and Embryo Transfer," p. 50.

109. Daniel Callahan, "Surrogate Motherhood: A Bad Idea," Editorial, *New York Times*, January 20, 1987, p. 25.

110. Paul Ramsey, "Shall We Reproduce?" p. 1349.

111. Gary B. Ellis, Office of Technology Assessment. Presentation at University of Virginia Reproductive Sciences Seminar Series, May 6, 1988.

112. Hans A. Tiefel, "Human In Vitro Fertilization," p. 3238. See also EAB, *Report and Conclusions*, p. 37, for a description of the belief that IVF "reflects an undue emphasis on the importance of biological parenthood." And Paul Ramsey, "Gruesome Futures," p. 41, in Jerome Lejeune and Paul Ramsey, eds., *The Question of In Vitro Fertilization*.

113. Robert H. Blank, *Rationing Medicine*, pp. 226–228.

114. *Ibid.*, p. 247, citing H. Tristam Engelhardt, Jr., and Michael A. Rie, "Intensive Care Units, Scarce Resources, and Conflicting Principles of Justice," *Journal of the American Medical Association* (1986), 255:1159–1164.

115. Quoted in Susan Abramowitz, "A Stalemate on Test-Tube Baby Research," p. 6.

116. Blank, *Rationing Medicine*, p. 80.

117. *Ibid.*, pp. 6, 249.

118. *Hearings on Embryo Transfer*, p. 32.

119. Andrea L. Bonnicksen and Robert H. Blank, "The Government and In Vitro Fertilization (IVF)."

120. Abramowitz, "Stalemate," p. 8; "A Once and Future Biomedical Ethics Board," p. 3.

121. See, for example, R. R. Angell, A. A. Templeton, and I. E. Messinis, "Consequences of Polyspermy in Man."

122. See, for example, J. L. Watt et al., "Trisomy 1 In An Eight Cell Human Pre-Embryo."

123. LeRoy Walters, "Ethics and New Reproductive Technologies: An International Review of Committee Statements," pp. 6S–7S.

124. Abramowitz, "Stalemate," p. 9.

125. Singer, "Australian Developments."

126. Office of Technology Assessment, *Infertility: Medical and Social Choices*, p. 298. But see VLA Secretariat, "The Third Report of the Voluntary Licensing Authority for Human *In Vitro* Fertilisation and Embryology," pp. 15, 28, for a study conducted to test the safety of egg freezing.

127. John A. Robertson, "The Law of Institutional Review Boards," p. 895.

128. See Robertson, "Scientist's Right to Research," p. 1277, who notes that federal funding is "an effective, though limited, tool for regulating scientific research."

129. For a discussion of each application, see CIBA Foundation, *Human Embryo Research; Yes or No?* pp. 66, 65, 72, and 122–136, respectively.

130. "Public Perceptions of And Support for Biotechnology," *Biolaw* (August 1987), p. U:552.

131. See Bonnicksen, "Advocacy of Human Embryo Research: Emerging Values."

132. John A. Robertson, "Embryo Research," pp. 17, 37; *Hearings on Embryo Transfer,* p. 264 (testimony of Richard P. Marrs); Robertson, "Ethical and Legal Issues in Cryopreservation of Human Embryos," p. 378; and Robertson, "Embryo Research," pp. 16–17.

133. *Hearings on Embryo Transfer,* p. 41 (testimony of Howard W. Jones, Jr.).

134. Robertson, "Embryo Research," p. 37.

135. CIBA Foundation, *Embryo Research,* p. 73.

136. "Embryo Research," Editorial, *Lancet* (February 2, 1985), 8423:255.

137. Robertson, *Embryo Research,* pp. 17, 27, 31; CIBA Foundation, *Embryo Research,* p. 74.

138. J. D. Schulman et al., "Genetic Aspects of IVF," in Christopher M. Fredericks et al., *Foundations of In Vitro Fertilization,* p. 199.

139. See, for example, W. French Anderson, "Human Gene Therapy: Scientific and Ethical Considerations," p. 290.

140. For a discussion, see Robertson, "Embryo Research."

141. In *Hearings on Embryo Transfer,* p. 146, for example, John Robertson, a law professor, said of the new conception techniques that they "[fall] squarely within constitutionally protected traditions of procreative liberty."

142. *Meyer v. Nebraska,* 262 U.S. 390 (1923); *Pierce v. Society of Sisters,* 268 U.S. 510 (1925); *Skinner v. Oklahoma,* 316 U.S. 535 (1942); *Griswold v. Connecticut,* 381 U.S. 479 (1965); *Eisenstadt v. Baird,* 405 U.S. 438 (1972); and, *Roe v. Wade,* 410 U.S. 113 (1973) and subsequent abortion decisions.

143. *Skinner v. Oklahoma,* 316 U.S. 535 (1942). Twenty-three years later, in striking down a Connecticut statute forbidding the use of birth control devices, Justice Douglas noted that the Court dealt with the sanctity of marriage and "a right of privacy older than the Bill of Rights." He went on to ask, "Would we allow the police to search the sacred precincts of marital bedrooms for telltale signs of the use of contraceptives? The very idea is repulsive to the notions of privacy surrounding the marriage relationship." *Griswold v. Connecticut,* 381 U.S. 479 (1965).

144. *Eisenstadt v. Baird,* 405 U.S. 438 (1972).

145. *Roe v. Wade,* 410 U.S. 113 (1973).

146. Albert Gore, Jr., speaking before Congress. *Congressional Record* (November 17, 1983) 129, No. 160, Part II, 98th Congress, 1st Session H10292.

147. Quoted in Sulzner, "Policy Process," p. 440.

148. Mendeloff, "Politics and Bioethical Commissions," pp. 85–86.

149. See Abram and Wolf, "Involvement," p. 627.

150. Quoted in Sulzner, "Policy Process," pp. 441–442.

151. Krause, "Artificial Conception," p. 193.
152. Abram and Wolf, "Public Involvement," p. 628.
153. *Ibid.*, pp. 628–629; *Hearings on Embryo Transfer.*
154. Abram and Wolf, "Public Involvement," p. 628.
155. Prepared statement of Gary B. Ellis, *Hearings on Consumer Protection Issues*, p. 12.
156. Walters, "Ethics and New Reproductive Technologies," p. 9S.
157. Robertson, "Scientist's Right to Research," p. 1278.

6. A RESPONSIBLE PUBLIC

1. A. Trounson and L. Mohr, "Human Pregnancy Following Cryopreservation, Thawing and Transfer of an Eight-Cell Embryo"; "First Baby Born of Frozen Embryo," *New York Times*, April 11, 1984, p. 14; and Peter Singer and Deane Wells, *The Reproductive Revolution: New Ways of Making Babies*, p. 99.

2. For a history of oocyte donations see Zev Rosenwaks et al., "Pregnancy Following Transfer of In Vitro Fertilized *Donated* Oocytes," *Fertility and Sterility* (March 1986), 45:417–420.

3. Maria Bustillo et al., "Delivery of a Healthy Infant Following Nonsurgical Ovum Transfer"; Maria Bustillo et al., "Nonsurgical Ovum Transfer as a Treatment in Infertile Women."

4. "Dear Abby," News Syndicate, November 28, 1986.

5. John D. Battersby, "Woman Pregnant with Daughter's Triplets," *New York Times*, April 9, 1987, p. 1; John D. Battersby, "South Africa Woman Gives Birth to 3 Grandchildren, and History," *New York Times*, October 2, 1987, p. A9.

6. *In the Matter of Baby M*, No. FM-25314-86E (Bergen County, N.J. Supreme Court, March 31, 1987); 13 F.L.R. 2001, April 7, 1987.

7. Transcript excerpts, reprinted in *New York Times*, February 5, 1987, p. 15.

8. Burke Breathed, Bloom County, *St. Louis Post-Dispatch*, April 26, 1987.

9. See, for example, Alexander Morgan Capron, "The New Reproductive Possibilities: Seeking a Moral Basis for Concerted Action in a Pluralistic Society," p. 194.

10. David Horsey, *Seattle Post-Intelligencer*, March 15, 1987.

11. *Chicago Tribune*, April 9, 1987, p. 18.

12. Andrew C. Varga, *The Main Issues in Bioethics*, rev. ed. (New York: Paulist Press, 1984), p. 1. See also Samuel Gorovitz, "Engineering Human Reproduction: A Challenge to Public Policy," p. 267: "Ethical issues center on questions of how people ought to treat one another."

13. Michael S. Gregory, "Science and Humanities: Toward a New World View," in D. Heyward Brock, ed., *The Culture of Biomedicine: Studies in Science and Culture*, 1:29.

14. See, for example, Strachan Donnelley, "Introduction to Biomedical Eth-

ics: A Multinational View," *Hastings Center Report* (June 1987), 17:2: "The more we technologically change things, the more they humanly stay the same." And see A. George Schillinger, "Man's Enduring Technological Dilemma."

15. Edmund D. Pellegrino, *Humanism and the Physician*, p. 13.

16. These titles appeared in the British press. R. G. Edwards and Peter Steptoe, *A Matter of Life*, p. 100.

17. Paul Ramsey, "The Issues Facing Mankind," in Jerome Lejeune and Paul Ramsey, *The Question of In Vitro Fertilization*, p. 21.

18. Paul Ramsey, "Shall We Reproduce?" p. 1346.

19. Letter to Editor, *British Medical Journal* (May 22, 1982), 284:1560.

20. Hans O. Tiefel, "Human In Vitro Fertilization: A Conservative View," p. 3242; Letter to Editor, *British Medical Journal* (June 25, 1982), 284:1950–1951; Letter to Editor, *British Medical Journal* (May 22, 1982), 284:1560.

21. Letter to Editor, *British Medical Journal* (June 25, 1982), 284:1950–1951. But see George J. Annas, testifying at *Hearings on Human Embryo Transfer*, p. 216: "we need more than a moral revulsion to legislate."

22. Eileen P. Flynn, *Human Fertilization In Vitro: A Catholic Moral Perspective*, p. 10. The countervailing argument, also reached on the basis of natural law, is that IVF "is designed to help human persons who want to realize a very basic human good" (p. 11). See also Letter to Editor, *British Medical Journal* (May 22, 1982), 284:1560.

23. See, for example, *Rochin v. California*, 342 U.S. 165 (1952).

24. "Instruction on Respect for Human Life in Its Origin and on the Dignity of Procreation: Replies to Certain Questions of the Day." Reprinted in *New York Times*, March 11, 1987, pp. 10–13.

25. Quoted in Letter to Editor, *British Medical Journal* (1982), 285:1114. See also "Hi-Tech in Eden," *Ethics and Medics* (August 1986), 11:1–2. For an opposite point of view, see Robert Francoeur, a Catholic philosopher, who said that of course humans could not take over God's role as creator. It was a "waste of time and energy for scientists, ethicists, and laymen alike to beat their breasts" over the question. Quoted in Gerald S. Snyder, *Test-Tube Life: Scientific Advance and Moral Dilemma* (New York: Julian Messner, 1982), p. 120.

26. Flynn, *Human Fertilization*, p. 4. See also Letter to Editor, *British Medical Journal* (October 16, 1982), 285:1115.

27. Flynn, *Human Fertilization*, p. 3, quoting from Psalms 127:3–5.

28. Mary Warnock, *A Question of Life: The Warnock Report on Human Fertilisation and Embryology*, p. 2.

29. *Ibid.*, p. 3.

30. Edwards and Steptoe, *Matter of Life*, p. 48.

31. Letter to Editor, *Nature*, January 24, 1985, 313:262.

32. Amitai Etzioni, *Genetic Fix*, p. 78, quoting Leon R. Kass.

33. Ramsey, "Issues," p. 26; Ramsey, "Reproduce?" p. 1349. For another account of the effects of new conceptions on the family, see Sidney Callahan,

"The Ethical Challenge of the New Reproductive Technology." And Ramsey, "Reproduce?" p. 1482, quoting Leon R. Kass.

34. See Tiefel, "Human IVF," p. 3236, for a description of this concern. See also Singer and Wells, *Reproductive Revolution*, p. 73; "Instruction on Respect for Human Life."

35. Flynn, *Human Fertilization*, p. 10, quoting Theodore Hall.

36. Ramsey, "Reproduce?" p. 1482, quoting Leon R. Kass. See also statements by Pope Pius XII at the Fourth International Congress of Catholic Doctors, September 29, 1949, on artificial insemination by donor (AID), in which he said that the dignity of marriage and the child's happiness depend upon procreation occuring "according to the will and plan of the Creator." See Snyder, *Test-Tube Life*, p. 116.

37. The group, formed in 1984, has held international meetings, including a conference in 1985 at which a resolution was passed that, among other things, called on women to "resist the take-over of our bodies for male use, for profit-making, population control, medical experimentation, and misogynous science." *Resolution of the Women's Emergency Conference on the New Reproductive Technologies* (1985).

38. Ruth Hubbard, "Personal Courage Is Not Enough: Some Hazards of Childbearing in the 1980s," in Rita Arditti et al., eds., *Test Tube Women*, p. 350.

39. Mary Anne Warren, *Gendercide: The Implications of Sex Selection*, p. 444; Jalna Hanmer, "A Womb of One's Own," in Arditti et al., eds., *Test Tube Women*, pp. 445, 438, and 444; Hubbard, "Courage," p. 350; and Alan L. Otten, "Artificial Birth Methods Are Attacked by Some Feminists Fearing Male Control," *Wall Street Journal*, May 1, 1986, p. 35.

40. Genoveffa Corea, "Egg Snatchers," in Arditti et al., eds., *Test Tube Women*, p. 45.

41. Margaret Atwood, *The Handmaid's Tale*, pp. 136, 73, and 74.

42. For a discussion of the embryo's value, see "Instruction"; and Letter to Editor, *Nature*, March 7, 1984, 314:10.

43. Jerome Lejeune, "Test Tube Babies *Are* Babies," in Lejeune and Ramsey, *Question of IVF*, p. 9.

44. Letter to Editor, *Nature*, March 7, 1984, 314:10. The embryo is a "distinct entity with all the necessary genetic attributes for being able to learn to read and write among any other endowments humans may have." National Council of the Society for the Protection of Unborn Children, "Man's Intrusion on Nature," in Lejeune and Ramsey, *Question of IVF*, p. 63. See also D. Gareth Jones, *Brave New People: Ethical Issues at the Commencement of Life*, p. 119.

45. National Council, "Man's Intrusion," pp. 62–63.

46. Letter to Editor, *Nature*, January 24, 1985, 313:262. See also Tiefel, "Human IVF," p. 3240, for the view that the embryo is life.

47. See, for example, the comments of Joseph Fletcher in Gebhard F. B. Schumacher et al., "In Vitro Fertilization of Human Ova and Blastocyst Trans-

fer," pp. 198–199; and J. Fletcher, "Ethical Aspects of Genetic Controls: Designed Genetic Changes in Man," *New England Journal of Medicine* (1971), 285:776–783.

48. See, for example, Flynn, *Human Fertilization*, p. 130.

49. *New York Times*, January 28, 1987, p. 19.

50. H. W. Jones, Jr., "The Ethics of In-Vitro Fertilization—1981," in R. G. Edwards and Jean M. Purdy, *Human Conception In Vitro*, p. 355.

51. This is even more puzzling when contrasted with events in China, where the one-child policy, if carried out to the letter, would do away with an entire group of relatives—sisters and brothers, nieces and nephews, aunts and uncles —all at once. In the Western hemisphere science has created new groups of relatives—gestational mothers, genetic mothers, social mothers, and surrogate mother/grandmothers—also all at once.

52. Jonathan Glover, *Causing Death and Saving Lives* (New York: Penguin Books, 1977), p. 289.

53. P. C. Steptoe and R. G. Edwards, "Reimplantation of a Human Embryo with Subsequent Tubal Pregnancy." But see Patrick Steptoe and Robert Edwards, "Pregnancy in an Infertile Patient After Transfer of an Embryo Fertilised in Vitro," Letter to Editor, *British Medical Journal* (April 23, 1983), 286:1351, for a letter in which the authors expressed concern with the implications of ovum transfer for women.

54. Sherman Elias and George J. Annas, "Social Policy Considerations in Noncoital Reproduction"; Clifford Grobstein et al., "External Human Fertilization: An Evaluation of Policy"; National Conference of Commissioners on Uniform State Laws, "Status of Children of the New Biology," draft report, 1987; Lori B. Andews, *New Conceptions: A Consumer's Guide to the Newest Infertility Treatment;* and *Warnock, Question of Life.*

55. Leon R. Kass, "Making Babies—The New Biology and the 'Old' Morality."

56. "Baby in a Bottle," *Science News* (July 22, 1978), 114:51; Pamela McCorduck, "Babies from the Lab," *Redbook*, June 1981, 157:31–33 + ; and K. S. Jayaraman, "India Reveals Deep-Frozen Test-Tube Baby," *New Scientist* (October 19, 1978), 80:159.

57. For the distinction between prepositions and nouns and adjectives in the naming process, I am indebted to Irving Zola of Brandeis University, and to the paper he read at the *Hastings Center, Briarcliff Manor, N.Y., October 16, 1987.*

58. *Benson, The Arizona Republic,* 1984 Tribune Media Services.

59. Mike Peters, *Dayton Daily News;* reprinted in *Charleston Times-Courier,* July 3, 1984, p. A4.

60. Hans Jonas, "Philosophical Aspects of Technology," *The Connecticut Scholar* (Occasional Papers of the Connecticut Humanities Council, 1980), p. 13.

61. Mother Goose & Grimm, 1984 Tribune Media Services.

62. Bennett, *St. Petersburg Times,* 1983 Copley News Service.

63. From Sybille Bedford, *Aldous Huxley: A Biography* (New York: Knopf/ Harper & Row, 1974), p. 245.

64. Corea, "Egg Snatchers," in Arditti et al., eds., *Test Tube Women*, pp. 37– 51, 41. Emphasis added.

65. Etzioni, *Genetic Fix*, pp. 19–56, emphasis added; and Jo Thomas, "British Debate Embryo Research," *New York Times*, October 16, 1984, p. C6, emphasis added.

66. Theodore Roszak, quoted in Dorothy Nelkin, "Science as a Source of Political Conflict," in Torgny Segerstedt, ed., *Ethics for Science Policy: Proceedings* (Elmsford, NY: Pergamon Press, 1979), p. 9.

67. Joyce Carol Oates, "A Terrible Beauty Is Born. How?" *New York Times Book Review* (August 11, 1985), p. 1.

68. A gynecologist testifying in the Del Zio trial. He said that with external fertilization, the embryo need not be subject to the four- to five-day trip down the fallopian tubes, which was an "extremely tortuous passage" whereby the embryo was "squeezed and forced." Judith Cummings, "Physician Testifies on 'Test-Tube Baby,' " *New York Times*, July 25, 1978, p. B3.

69. Quoted in *New York Times Book Review*, September 1, 1985, p. 3.

70. Glover, *Causing Death*, p. 288.

71. Jeremy Rifkin, *Declaration of a Heretic*, p. 41. He was referring to the change from the "Age of Pyrotechnology to the Age of Biotechnology."

72. Brendan Gill, "Still Here at the New Yorker," *New York Times Book Review*, October 4, 1987, p. 37.

73. "Ethics in Embryo," *Harper's Magazine* (September 1987), pp. 37–47.

74. Leon R. Kass, *Toward a More Natural Science*, p. 100.

75. See, for example, Helen Bequaert Holmes and Tjeerd Tymstra, "In Vitro Fertilization in the Netherlands: Experiences and Opinions of Dutch Women"; Patsy Littlejohn, "IVF Patients and their Attitudes to Ethical Issues: Replies to a Questionnaire," in Singer and Wells, *Reproductive Revolution*, pp. 234–247.

76. LeRoy Walters, "Ethics and New Reproductive Technologies."

77. Andrea Bonnicksen, "Advocacy of Human Embryo Research," p. S92.

78. Nelkin, "Science as a Source," in Segersredt, ed., *Ethics*, p. 9, 22.

7. LOOKING TO THE FUTURE

1. Daniel Callahan, "Ethics and Recombinant DNA Research," *The Connecticut Scholar* (Occasional Papers of the Connecticut Humanities Council, 1980), p. 57.

2. George Lakoff and Mark Johnson, "Conceptual Metaphors in Everyday Language."

3. George Orwell, "Politics and the English Language," *The Norton Anthology of English Literature*, 5th ed., (New York: Norton, 1986), 2:2262.

4. Philip L. Bereano, "Courts as Institutions for Assessing Technology," in Williams A. Thomas, ed., *Scientists in the Legal System*, p. 77, quoting Oliver Wendell Holmes.

5. Quoted in Robyn Rowland, "Making Women Visible in the Embryo Experimentation Debate," p. 182.

6. Alistair V. Campbell, *Moral Dilemmas in Medicine*, p. 6.

7. Hans Jonas, "Philosophical Aspects of Technology," *The Connecticut Scholar* (Occasional Papers of the Connecticut Humanities Council, 1980), p. 10.

8. Carl Sagan, "The Role of Science and Technology," p. 51.

9. Edmund Pellegrino, "The Anatomy of Clinical Ethical Judgments in Perinatology and Neonatology."

10. See, for example, Peter Singer and Helga Kuhse, "The Ethics of Embryo Research"; Hans-Martin Sass, "Moral Dilemmas in Perinatal Medicine and the Quest for Large Scale Embryo Research: A Discussion of Recent Guidelines in the Federal Republic of Germany."

11. Transcript of tape-recorded conversation, p. 11.

APPENDIX

1. Peter Roberts, "The Brennan Story: A Small Miracle of Creation," in William A. W. Walters and Peter Singer, eds., *Test-Tube Babies*, p. 12.

2. P. C. Steptoe and J. Webster, "Laparoscopy of the Normal and Disordered Ovary," in R. G. Edwards and Jean M. Purdy, *Human Conception In Vitro*, p. 101.

3. Edwards and Purdy, *Human Conception*, p. 35; J. Cohen et al., "Endocrinology of the Menstrual Cycle with Reference to Fertilization *In Vitro*," in Edwards and Purdy, *Human Conception*, p. 15.

4. Steptoe and Webster, in Edwards and Purdy, *Human Conception*, p. 100.

5. Edwards and Purdy, *Human Conception*, p. 87.

6. Roberts, "Brennan Story," p. 12.

7. *Ibid.*

8. Steptoe and Webster, in Edwards and Purdy, *Human Conception*, p. 101.

9. Roberts, "Brennan Story," p. 12.

10. Edwards and Purdy, *Human Conception*, p. 87.

11. Roberts, "Brennan Story," p. 13.

12. Steptoe and Webster, in Edwards and Purdy, *Human Conception*, p. 101.

13. Roberts, "Brennan Story," p. 13.

14. Machelle M. Seibel, "A New Era in Reproductive Technology," p. 829.

15. See Seibel, pp. 829–830, for a description of types.

16. J. Mandelbaum et al., "The Use of Clomid and hMG in Human In Vitro Fertilization: Consequences for Egg Quality and Luteal Phase Adequacy," in Henning M. Beier and Hans R. Lindner, eds., *Fertilization of the Human Egg In Vitro*, p. 124.

17. Roberts, "Brennan Story," p. 13.
18. Lucinda L. Veeck, *Atlas of the Human Oocyte and Early Conceptus.*
19. Seibel, "New Era," p. 830.
20. Albert Decker and Suzanne Loebl, *Why Can't We Have a Baby?* pp. 37–38.
21. Seibel, "New Era," p. 830.
22. Roberts, "Brennan Story," p. 16.
23. J. M. Purdy, "Methods for Fertilization and Embryo Culture *In Vitro*," in Edwards and Purdy, *Human Conception,* pp. 136, 141.
24. For a discussion of water quality and IVF, see Judy Fleetham and Maha M. Mahadevan, "Purification of Water for In Vitro Fertilization and Embryo Transfer," *Journal of In Vitro Fertilization and Embryo Transfer* (June 1988), 5:171–174.
25. Roberts, "Brennan Story," p. 16.
26. L. R. Mohr et al., "Evaluation of Normal and Abnormal Human Embryo Development During Procedures In Vitro," in Beier and Lindner, *Fertilization,* pp. 211–221.
27. Seibel, "New Era," pp. 830–831.

Selected Bibliography

Abram, Morris B. and Susan M. Wolf. "Public Involvement in Medical Ethics." *New England Journal of Medicine* (March 8, 1984), 310:627–632.

Abramowitz, Susan. "A Stalemate on Test-Tube Baby Research." *Hastings Center Report* (February 1984), 14:5–9.

Adler, Elizabeth M. et al. "Attitudes of Women of Reproductive Age to *In Vitro* Fertilization and Embryo Research." *Journal of Biosocial Science* (April 1986), 18:155–167.

Adler, Elizabeth M. and A. A. Templeton. "Patient Reaction to IVF Treatment." Letter to Editor. *Lancet* (January 19, 1985), 1:8421:168.

American Association for the Advancement of Science. "Resolution on Reestablishment of the Ethics Advisory Board, U.S. Department of Health and Human Services." May 29, 1986.

American Fertility Society. "New Guidelines for the Use of Semen Donor Insemination: 1986." *Fertility and Sterility* (October 1986), 46:95S–110S.

Anderson, W. French. "Human Gene Therapy: Scientific and Ethical Considerations." *Journal of Medicine and Philosophy* (August 1985), 10:275–291.

Anderson, W. French and John C. Fletcher. "Gene Therapy in Human Beings: When Is It Ethical to Begin?" *New England Journal of Medicine* (November 27, 1980), 303:1293–1297.

Andrews, Lori B. "Legal and Ethical Aspects of New Reproductive Technologies." *Clinical Obstetrics and Gynecology* (March 1986), 29:190–204.

—— *New Conceptions: A Consumer's Guide to the Newest Infertility Treatment.* New York: St. Martin's Press, 1984.

—— "The Stork Market: The Law of the New Reproductive Technologies." *American Bar Association Journal* (August 1984), 70:50–56.

Angell, Roslyn R., A. A. Templeton, and R. J. Aitken. "Chromosomal Studies in Human In Vitro Fertilization." *Human Genetics* (1986), 72:333–339.

Angell, Roslyn R., A. A. Templeton, and I. E. Messinis. "Consequences of Polyspermy in Man." *Cytogenetics Cell Genetics* (1986), 42:1–7.

Angell, Roslyn R. et al. "Chromosomal Abnormalities in Human Embryos After *In Vitro* Fertilization" *Nature*, May 26, 1983, 303:336–338.

Annas, George J. "Making Babies Without Sex: The Law and the Profits." *American Journal of Public Health* (December 1984), 74:1415–1417.

—— "Redefining Parenthood and Protecting Embryos: Why We Need New Laws." *Hastings Center Report* (October 1984), 14:50–52.

Annas, George J. and Sherman Elias. "*In Vitro* Fertilization and Embryo Transfer: Medicolegal Aspects of New Techniques to Create a Family." *Family Law Quarterly* (Summer 1983), 17:199–223.

Aral, Sevgi O. et al. "The Increasing Concern with Infertility: Why Now?" *Journal of the American Medical Association* (November 4, 1983), 250:2327–2331.

Arditti, Rita, Renate Duelli Klein, and Shelly Minden, eds. *Test Tube Women.* London: Pandora Press, 1984.

Atwood, Margaret. *The Handmaid's Tale.* Boston: Houghton Mifflin, 1986.

"Baby Craving." *Life*, June 1987, pp. 36–42.

Batterman, Ronni. "A Comprehensive Approach to Treating Infertility." *Health and Social Work* (Winter 1985), 10:46–54.

Battersby, John D. "Woman Pregnant with Daughter's Triplets." *New York Times*, April 9, 1987, p. 1.

Beauchamp, Tom L. and James F. Childress. *Principles of Biomedical Ethics.* 2d ed. New York: Oxford University Press, 1983.

Beier, Henning M. and Hans R. Lindner, eds. *Fertilization of the Human Egg In Vitro.* Berlin: Springer-Verlag, 1983.

Bernstein, Judith et al. "Assessment of Psychological Dysfunction Associated with Infertility." *Journal of Obstetrics, Gynecology and Neonatal Nursing* (November/December 1985), 14:63S–66S.

Blackwell, Richard E. et al. "Are We Exploiting the Infertile Couple?" *Fertility and Sterility* (November 1987), 48:735–739.

Blakeslee, Sandra. "Trying to Make Money Making 'Test-Tube' Babies." *New York Times*, May 17, 1987, p. 6, s. 6.

Blank, Robert H. "Making Babies: The State of the Art." *The Futurist* (February 1985), 19:11–17.

—— *Rationing Medicine.* New York: Columbia University Press, 1988.

Bonnicksen, Andrea L. "Advocacy of Human Embryo Research: Emerging Values." *BioLaw* (March 1988), 2:S:91–S:100.

—— "In Vitro Fertilization and Public Policy: Turning to the Consumer." *Population Research and Policy Review* (1986), 5:197–215.

Bonnicksen, Andrea L. and Robert H. Blank. "The Government and In Vitro

Fertilization (IVF): Views of IVF Directors." *Fertility and Sterility* (March 1988), 49:396–398.

Brahams, Diana. "In Vitro Fertilization and Related Research: Why Parliament Must Legislate." *Lancet* (September 24, 1983), 2:8352:726–729.

Brock, D. Heyward, ed. *The Culture of Biomedicine: Studies in Science and Culture*, Vol. 1. Newark: University of Delaware Press, 1984.

Brody, Eugene B. "Reproduction Without Sex—But with the Doctor." *Law, Medicine & Health Care* (Fall 1987), 15:152–155.

Brotman, Harris. "Human Embryo Transplants." *New York Times Magazine*, January 8, 1984, pp. 42–49.

Brumby, Margaret and Pascal Kasimba. "When Is Cloning Lawful?" *Journal of In Vitro Fertilization and Embryo Transfer* (August 1987), 4:198–204.

Buster, John E. et al. "Non-Surgical Transfer of an In-Vivo Fertilised Donated Ovum to an Infertility Patient." *Lancet* (April 9, 1983), 1:8328:816–817.

Bustillo, Maria et al. "Delivery of a Healthy Infant Following Nonsurgical Ovum Transfer." Letter to Editor. *Journal of the American Medical Association* (February 17, 1984), 251:889.

—— et al. "Nonsurgical Ovum Transfer as a Treatment in Infertile Women." *Journal of the American Medical Association* (March 2, 1984), 251:1171–1173.

Callahan, Daniel. "Contemporary Biomedical Ethics." *New England Journal of Medicine* (1980), 302:1228–1233.

Callahan, Sidney. "The Ethical Challenge of the New Reproductive Technology." In David Thomasma and John Monagle, eds. *Medical Ethics: A Guide for Health Professionals*. Rockville, Md.: Aspen, 1988.

Campagnoli, C. et al. "Patient Selection for In Vitro Fertilization (IVF) and Embryo Transfer (ET)." *Experientia*, December 15, 1985, 41:1491–1494.

Campbell, Alistair V. *Moral Dilemmas in Medicine*. Baltimore: Williams & Wilkins, 1972.

Capron, Alexander Morgan. "The New Reproductive Possibilities: Seeking a Moral Basis for Concerted Action in a Pluralistic Society." *Law, Medicine & Health Care* (October 1984), 12:192–198.

Cardozo, Benjamin N. *The Paradoxes of Legal Science*. Westport, Conn.: Greenwood Press, 1956.

Chillick, Claudio F. "The Role of In Vitro Fertilization in Infertile Patients with Endometriosis." *Fertility and Sterility* (July 1985), 44:56–61.

Christie, G. L. "The Psychological and Social Management of the Infertile Couple." In R. J. Pepperell et al., eds. *The Infertile Couple*, pp. 229–247. London: Churchill Livingstone, 1980.

CIBA Foundation. *Human Embryo Research: Yes or No?* London: Tavistock, 1986.

Clapp, Diane. "Emotional Responses to Infertility." *Journal of Obstetrics, Gynecology, and Neonatal Nursing* (November/December 1985), 14:32S–35S.

Committee on Ethics. American College of Obstetricians and Gynecologists.

179

Selected Bibliography

"ACOG Committee Statement: Ethical Issues on Human In Vitro Fertilization and Embryo Placement." 1986.

Committee on Gynecologic Practice. American College of Obstetricians and Gynecologists. "ACOG Committee Statement: Human In Vitro Fertilization and Embryo Placement." 1984.

Corea, Gena. *The Mother Machine: Reproductive Technologies from Artificial Insemination to Artificial Wombs.* New York: Harper and Row, 1985.

—— "Unnatural Selection." *The Progressive* (January 1986), 50:22–24.

Corea, Gena et al. *Man-Made Women: How New Reproductive Technologies Affect Women.* Bloomington: Indiana University Press, 1987.

Crabtree, Ellen. "Protecting Inheritance Rights of Children Born Through *In Vitro* Fertilization and Embryo Transfer: Suggestions for a Legislative Approach." *Saint Louis University Law Journal* (November 1983), 27:901–928.

Davis, Gwen. "The Private Pain of Infertility." *New York Times Magazine,* December 6, 1987, pp. 104+.

DeCherney, Alan H. "Doctored Babies." *Fertility and Sterility* (December 1983), 20:724–727.

Decker, Albert and Suzanne Loebl. *Why Can't We Have a Baby?* New York: Dial Press, 1978.

Department of Health and Social Security. "Legislation on Human Infertility Services and Embryo Research: A Consultation Paper." London: Her Majesty's Stationery Office, 1986.

"Draft Legislation on Infertility Services and Embryo Research." *Lancet* (December 5, 1987), 2:8571:1343.

Eagan, Andrea Boroff. "Baby Roulette." *The Village Voice,* August 25, 1987, pp. 16+.

Edwards, R. G. et al. "Factors Influencing the Success of In Vitro Fertilization for Alleviating Human Infertility." *Journal of In Vitro Fertilization and Embryo Transfer* (March 1984), 1:3–23.

Edwards, R. G. and Jean M. Purdy. *Human Conception In Vitro.* London: Academic Press, 1982.

Edwards, R. G. and Patrick Steptoe. *A Matter of Life.* New York: Morrow, 1980.

Edwards, R. G., P. C. Steptoe, and J. M. Purdy. "Fertilization and Cleavage In Vitro of Preovulator Human Oocytes." *Nature* (1970), 227:1307–1309.

Elias, Sherman and George J. Annas. "Social Policy Considerations in Noncoital Reproduction." *Journal of the American Medical Association* (January 3, 1986), 255:62–68.

Ellul, Jacques. *The Technological Society.* New York: Vintage Books, 1964.

"Embryo Research." Editorial. *Lancet* (February 2, 1985), 1:8423:255–256.

"Ethical Statement on In Vitro Fertilization." *Fertility and Sterility* (January 1984), 41:13.

Ethics Advisory Board. Department of Health, Education, and Welfare. *Appendix: HEW Support of Research Involving Human IN VITRO Fertilization and Embryo Transfer.* Washington, D.C.: GPO, May 4, 1979.

Ethics Advisory Board, Department of Health, Education, and Welfare. *Report and Conclusions: HEW Support of Research Involving Human In Vitro Fertilization and Embryo Transfer.* Washington, D.C.: GPO, May 4, 1979.

Ethics Committee of the American Fertility Society. "Ethical Considerations of the New Reproductive Technologies." *Fertility and Sterility* (September 1986), 46:1S–94S.

Ethics Committee (1986–1987) of the American Fertility Society. "Ethical Considerations of the New Reproductive Technologies in Light of Instruction on the Respect for Human Life in Its Origin and on Dignity of Procreation." *Fertility and Sterility* (February 1988), 49:1S–7S.

"Ethics in Embryo." *Harper's Magazine,* September 1987, pp. 37–47.

Etzioni, Amitai. *Genetic Fix.* New York: Macmillan, 1973.

Fletcher, John C. "Ethical Issues In and Beyond Prospective Clinical Trials of Human Gene Therapy." *Journal of Medicine and Philosophy* (August 1985), 10:293–309.

Fletcher, John C. and Kenneth J. Ryan. "Federal Regulations for Fetal Research: A Case for Reform." *Law, Medicine & Health Care* (Fall 1987), 15:126–138.

Fletcher, Joseph. *The Ethics of Genetic Control: Ending Reproductive Roulette.* Garden City, NY: Anchor Books, 1974.

Florman, Samuel C. *Blaming Technology: The Irrational Search for Scapegoats.* New York: St. Martin's Press, 1981.

Flynn, Eileen P. *Human Fertilization In Vitro: A Catholic Moral Perspective.* New York: University Press of America, 1984.

Formigli, Leonardo. "Donation of Fertilized Uterine Ova to Infertile Women." *Fertility and Sterility* (January 1987), 47:162–165.

Fredericks, Christopher M., John D. Paulson and Alan H. DeCherney, eds., *Foundations of In Vitro Fertilization* Washington, D.C.: Hemisphere Publishing, 1987.

Freeman, Ellen W. et. al. "Psychological Evaluation and Support in a Program of In Vitro Fertilization and Embryo Transfer." *Fertility and Sterility* (January 1985), 43:48–53.

"French Researcher Says 'Non' to Egg Manipulation." *Hastings Center Report* (December 1986), 16:4.

"Genetic Engineering in Man: Ethical Considerations." Editorial. *Journal of the American Medical Association* (May 1, 1972), 220:721.

Gorovitz, Samuel. "Engineering Human Reproduction: A Challenge to Public Policy." *Journal of Medicine and Philosophy* (August 1985), 10:267–274.

Greenfeld, Dorothy et al. "The Role of the Social Worker in the In-Vitro Fertilization Program." *Social Work in Health Care* (Winter 1984), 10:71–79.

Greenfeld, Dorothy and Florence Haseltine. "Candidate Selection and Psychosocial Considerations of In-Vitro Fertilization Procedures." *Clinical Obstetrics and Gynecology* (March 1986), 29:119–126.

Grobstein, Clifford. "The Early Development of Human Embryos." *Journal of Medicine and Philosophy* (August 1985), 10:213–236.

Selected Bibliography

—— From Chance to Purpose: An Appraisal of External Human Fertilization. Reading, Mass.: Addison-Wesley, 1981.

Grobstein, Clifford, Michael Flower and John Mendeloff. "External Human Fertilization: An Evaluation of Policy." *Science,* October 14, 1983, 222:127–133.

Grobstein, Clifford et al. "Frozen Embryos: Policy Issues." *New England Journal of Medicine* (June 13, 1985), 312:1584–1588.

Guttmacher, Alan F. "Early Attitudes Toward Infertility." *Proceedings of the First World Congress on Fertility and Sterility.* May 25–31, 1953, pp. 1–12.

Hammond, Mary G. and Luther M. Talbert. *Infertility: Practical Guide for the Physician.* 2d ed. Oradell, N.J.: Medical Economics Books, 1985.

Hanley, Robert. "Legislators Are Hesitant on Regulating Surrogacy." *New York Times,* February 4, 1988, p. B7.

Harrison, Keith L. et al. "Stress and Semen Quality in an In Vitro Fertilization Program." *Fertility and Sterility* (October 1987), 48:633–636.

Hayes, Maria F. "Effect of General Anesthesia on Fertilization and Cleavage of Human Oocytes In Vitro." *Fertility and Sterility* (December 1987), 48:975–981.

Hearings on Alternative Reproductive Technologies: Implications for Children and Families. U.S. Congress. House of Representatives. Select Committee on Children, Youth, and Families. 100th Congress. Washington, D.C.: GPO, 1987.

Hearings on Consumer Protection Issues Involving In Vitro Fertilization Clinics. U.S. Congress. House of Representatives. Committee on Small Business. Subcommittee on Regulation and Business Opportunities. 100th Congress. June 1, 1988 (prepublication materials).

Hearings on Human Embryo Transfer. U.S. Congress. House of Representatives. Committee on Science and Technology. Subcommittee on Investigations and Oversight. 98th Congress. 2nd Session. Washington, D.C.: GPO, 1985.

"Hi-Tech in Eden." *Ethics & Medics* (August 1986), 11:1–2.

Hodgkin, Paul. "Medicine Is War: And Other Medical Metaphors." *British Medical Journal* (December 21, 1985), 291:1820–1821.

Holmes, Helen Bequaert and Tjeerd Tymstra. "In Vitro Fertilization in the Netherlands: Experiences and Opinions of Dutch Women." *Journal of In Vitro Fertilization and Embryo Transfer* (1987), 4:116–123.

Hull, G. R. et al. "Population Study of Causes, Treatment, and Outcome of Infertility." *British Medical Journal* (December 14, 1985), 291:1693–1697.

"Human Embryo Research: Vote for Progress." *Lancet* (December 5, 1987), 2:8571:1311.

Huxley, Aldous. *Brave New World.* New York: Harper and Row, 1st Perennial Library Edition, 1969.

—— *Brave New World Revisited.* New York: Harper, 1958.

"Instruction on Respect for Human Life in Its Origin and on the Dignity of Procreation: Replies to Certain Questions of the Day." Doctrinal Statement of the Vatican. March 10, 1987.

Selected Bibliography

Jones, D. Gareth. *Brave New People: Ethical Issues at the Commencement of Life.* Downers Grove, Ill.: Inter-Varsity Press, 1984.

Jones, Howard W., Jr. "Variations on a Theme." Editorial. *Journal of the American Medical Association* (October 28, 1983), 250:2182–2183.

—— "The Process of Human Fertilization: Implications for Moral Status." *Fertility and Sterility* (August 1987), 48:189–192.

—— "What Is a Pregnancy? A Question for Programs of In Vitro Fertilization." *Fertility and Sterility* (December 1983), 40:728–733.

Kass, Leon R. "Ethical Dilemmas in the Care of the Ill. Part I. What Is the Physician's Service?" *Journal of the American Medical Association* (October 17, 1980), 244:1811–1816.

—— "Ethical Dilemmas in the Care of the Ill. Part II. What Is the Patient's Good?" *Journal of the American Medical Association* (October 24, 1980), 244:1946–1949.

—— "Making Babies—The New Biology and the 'Old' Morality." *Public Interest* (Winter 1972), 26:18–56.

—— *Toward a More Natural Science.* New York: Free Press, 1985.

Kemeter, Peter et al. "Psychosocial Testing and Pretreatment of Women for *In Vitro* Fertilization." *Annals of the New York Academy of Sciences* (1985), 442:523–532.

Kerin, John F. et al. "Incidence of Multiple Pregnancy After In-Vitro Fertilisation and Embryo Transfer." *Lancet* (September 3, 1983), 2:8349:537–540.

King, Patricia A. "Reproductive Technologies: Legal and Ethical Issues." *BioLaw* (1986), 1:113–148.

Kovacs, Gabor T. et al. "The Attitudes of the Australian Community to Treatment of Infertility by In Vitro Fertilization and Associated Procedures." *Journal of In Vitro Fertilization and Embryo Transfer* (1985), 2:213–216.

Krause, Harry D. "Artificial Conception: Legislative Approaches." *Family Law Quarterly* (Fall 1985), 19:185–206.

Lakoff, George and Mark Johnson. "Conceptual Metaphors in Everyday Language." *Journal of Philosophy* (August 1980), 77:453–486.

Leeton, John et al. "Pregnancy Established in an Infertile Patient After Transfer of an Embryo Fertilized in Vitro Where the Oocyte Was Donated by the Sister of the Recipient." *Journal of In Vitro Fertilization and Embryo Transfer* (1986), 3:379–382.

Leeton, John and Jayne Harman. "Attitudes Toward Egg Donation of Thirty-Four Infertile Women Who Donated During Their In Vitro Fertilization Treatment." *Journal of In Vitro Fertilization and Embryo Transfer* (1986), 3:374–378.

Lejeune, Jerome and Paul Ramsey, eds. *The Question of In Vitro Fertilization: Studies in Medicine, Law, and Ethics.* London: Society for the Protection of Unborn Children Educational Trust, 1984.

Lindsey, Robert. "Adoption Market: Big Demand, Tight Supply." *New York Times,* April 5, 1987, p. 1.

Lockwood, Michael, ed. *Moral Dilemmas in Modern Medicine.* New York: Oxford University Press, 1985.

Loevinger, Lee. "Science, Technology and Law in Modern Society." *Jurimetrics* (Fall 1985), 26:1–20.

Lyles, Rodney et al. "Characterization and Response of Women Undergoing Repeated Cycles of Ovulation Induction in an In Vitro Fertilization and Embryo Transfer Program." *Fertility and Sterility* (December 1985), 44:832–834.

Mahlstedt, Patricia and Linda D. Applegarth. "The Psychosocial Issues of In Vitro Fertilization: Coping and Control." *Abstracts of the 2nd Annual Conference for IVF Nurse Coordinators.* April 3–5, 1987.

Mao, K. and Carl Wood. "Decisions About the Use of Embryos." Letter to the Editor. *Lancet* (1983), 2:8362:1306–1307.

Mazor, Miriam D. and Harriet F. Simons, eds. *Infertility: Medical, Emotional and Social Considerations.* New York: Human Sciences Press, 1984.

McCormick, Rev. Richard A. "Ethics of Reproductive Technology: AFS Recommendations, Dissent." *Health Progress* (March 1987), pp. 33–37.

McLaren, Anne. "Prenatal Diagnosis Before Implantation: Opportunities and Problems." *Prenatal Diagnosis* (1985), 5:85–90.

—— "Research on Early Human Embryos from In-Vitro Fertilization (IVF): The Warnock Recommendations." *British Journal of Obstetrics and Gynecology* (April 1985), 92:305–307.

Medical Research Council and Royal College of Obstetricians and Gynaecologists. "The Second Report of the Voluntary Licensing Authority for Human *In Vitro* Fertilisation and Embryology." (April 1987).

Medical Research International. American Fertility Society Special Interest Group. "In Vitro Fertilization/Embryo Transfer in the United States: 1985 and 1986 Results from the National IVF/ET Registry." *Fertility and Sterility* (February 1988), 49:212–215.

Mendeloff, John. "Politics and Bioethical Commissions: 'Muddling Through' and the 'Slippery Slope.'" *Journal of Health Politics, Policy and Law* (Spring 1985), 10:81–92.

Menning, Barbara. *Infertility: A Guide for the Childless Couple.* Englewood Cliffs, N.J.: Prentice-Hall, 1977.

Merry, Sally Engle. "Concepts of Law and Justice Among Working-Class Americans: Ideology as Culture." *Legal Studies Forum* (1985), 9:59–69.

"Minimal Standards for Programs of In Vitro Fertilization." *Fertility and Sterility* (January 1984), 41:13.

National Perinatal Statistics Unit. *In Vitro Fertilization Pregnancies—Australia 1980–1983.* Sydney: Fertility Society of Australia, 1984.

National Perinatal Statistics Unit. Fertility Society of Australia. *In Vitro Fertilisation Pregnancies, Australia and New Zealand, 1979–1986.* Sydney: NPSU, 1987.

Nelkin, Dorothy. "Science as a Source of Political Conflict." In Torgny Segerstedt, ed. *Ethics for Science Policy: Proceedings*, pp. 9–24. Elmsford, NY: Pergamon Press, 1979.

Nero, Filomena A. and Alan H. DeCherney. The First Annual Conference of In Vitro Fertilization Nurse Coordinators." *Journal of In Vitro Fertilization and Embryo Transfer*. (1986), 3:277–278.

Note. "Reproductive Technology and the Procreation Rights of the Unmarried." *Harvard Law Review* (January 1985), 98:669–685.

Office for Protection from Research Risks. Office of the Director. National Institutes of Health. *Report on the Public Response to* In Vitro *Fertilization and Embryo Transfer*. April 15, 1980.

Office of Technology Assessment. U.S. Congress. *Infertility: Medical and Social Choices*. OTA-BA-358. Washington, D.C.: GPO, May 1988.

"A Once and Future Biomedical Ethics Board." *Hastings Center Report* (April/May 1988), 18:2–3.

Ontario Law Reform Commission. *Report on Human Artificial Reproduction and Related Matters*. Ontario: Ministry of the Attorney General, 1985.

Orwell, George. *1984*. New York: Harcourt Brace, 1949.

Otten, Alan L. "Artificial Birth Methods Are Attacked by Some Feminists Fearing Male Control." *Wall Street Journal*, May 1, 1986, p. 35.

—— "Infertility Enterprises Give Birth to Concern." *Wall Street Journal*, August 27, 1984, p. 12.

—— "Medical Efforts to Help Childless Couples Pose Host of Difficult Issues." *Wall Street Journal*, August 7, 1984, p. 1.

Ozar, David T. "The Case Against Thawing Unused Frozen Embryos." *Hastings Center Report* (August 1985), 15:7–12.

Palmiter, R. D. et al. "Dramatic Growth of Mice That Develop from Eggs Microinjected with Metallothionein-Growth Hormone Fusion Genes." *Nature* (1982), 301:611–615.

Pellegrino, Edmund D. *Humanism and the Physician*. Knoxville: University of Tennessee Press, 1979.

—— "The Anatomy of Clinical-Ethical Judgments in Perinatology and Neonatology: A Substantive and Procedural Framework." *Seminars in Perinatology* (July 1987), 11:202–209.

—— "Toward a Reconstruction of Medical Morality: The Primacy of the Act of Profession and the Fact of Illness." *Journal of Medicine and Philosophy* (1979), 4:32–56.

Plachot, Michelle et al. "From Oocyte to Embryo: A Model, Deduced from In Vitro Fertilization, for Natural Selection Against Chromosome Abnormalities." *Annales de Génétique (Paris)* (1987), 30:22–32.

"Public Perceptions of And Support for Biotechnology." *BioLaw* (August 1987), U:551–552.

Quist, Norman. "Institutional Review Boards and Human Subjects Research." *Bioethics Reporter* (1984), 1:825–830.

Ramsey, Paul. *On In Vitro Fertilization*. Chicago: Americans United for Life, n.d.

—— "Shall We 'Reproduce'?" *Journal of the American Medical Association* (June 5, 1972), 220:1346–1350; and (June 12, 1972), 220: 1480–1485.

"Recommendations of the Warnock Committee." *Lancet* (July 28, 1984), 2:8346:217–218.

"Report of the Royal College of Obstetricians and Gynaecologists on In Vitro Fertilisation and Embryo Replacement." *British Medical Journal* (May 7, 1983), 286:1519.

Rifkin, Jeremy. *Declaration of a Heretic.* Boston: Routledge and Kegan Paul, 1985.

Robertson, John A. "Embryo Research." *University of Western Ontario Law Review* (1986), 24:15–37.

—— "Embryos, Families, and Procreative Liberty: The Legal Structure of the New Reproduction." *Southern California Law Review* (1986), 59:939–1041.

—— "Ethical and Legal Issues in Cryopreservation of Human Embryos." *Fertility and Sterility* (March 1987), 47:371–381.

—— "Procreative Liberty and the Control of Conception, Pregnancy, and Childbirth." *Virginia Law Review* (April 1983), 69:405–464.

—— "The Law of Institutional Review Boards." *Bioethics Reporter* (1984), 1:832–897.

—— "The Scientist's Right to Research: A Constitutional Analysis." *Southern California Law Review* (1977–78), 51:1203–1279.

Romeu, Alberto et al. "Results of In Vitro Fertilization Attempts in Women 40 Years of Age and Older: The Norfolk Experience." *Fertility and Sterility* (January 1987), 47:130–136.

Rosenwaks, B. V. et al. "Pregnancy Following Transfer of Fertilized *Donated* Oocytes." *Fertility and Sterility* (March 1986), 45:417–420.

Rowland, Robyn. "Making Women Visible in the Embryo Experimentation Debate." *Bioethics* (April 1987), 1:179–188.

Sagan, Carl. "The Role of Science and Technology." *Current* (April 1977), 192:47–63.

Sass, Hans-Martin. "Moral Dilemmas in Perinatal Medicine and the Quest for Large Scale Embryo Research: A Discussion of Recent Guidelines in the Federal Republic of Germany." *Journal of Medicine and Philosophy* (August 1985), 10:279–290.

Schillinger, A. George. "Man's Enduring Technological Dilemma." *Technology in Society* (1984), 6:59–71.

Schumacher, Gebhard F. B. et al. "In Vitro Fertilization of Human Ova and Blastocyst Transfer: An Invitational Symposium." *Journal of Reproductive Medicine* (November 1973), 11:192–200.

Schauer, Frederick. "Slippery Slopes." *Harvard Law Review* (1985–1986), 99:361–383.

Scott, Russell. *The Body as Property.* New York: Viking, 1981.

Seibel, Machelle M. "A New Era in Reproductive Technology." *New England Journal of Medicine* (March 31, 1988), 318:828–834.

Shanahan, Louise. "In Vitro Fertilization." American Life Lobby, 1984.

Shettles, Landrum B. "A Morula Stage of Human Ovum Developed In Vitro." *Fertility and Sterility* (1955), 6:287–289.

—— *Ovum Humanum.* New York: Hafner, 1960.

Singer, Peter. "Australian Developments in Reproductive Technology." *Hastings Center Report* (April/May 1988), 18:4.

—— "Making Laws on Making Babies." *Hastings Center Report* (August 1985), 15:5–6.

Singer, Peter and Helga Kuhse. "The Ethics of Embryo Research." *Law, Medicine & Health Care* (September 1986), 14:133–137.

Singer, Peter and Deane Wells. *The Reproductive Revolution: New Ways of Making Babies.* Oxford University Press, 1984.

Smith, George P. II. "Australia's Frozen 'Orphan' Embryos: A Medical, Legal and Ethical Dilemma." *Journal of Family Law* (1985–1986), 24:27–41.

Soules, Michael R. "The In Vitro Fertilization Pregnancy Rate: Let's Be Honest with One Another." *Fertility and Sterility* (April 1985), 43:511–513.

Stanley, Manfred. *The Technological Conscience: Survival and Dignity in An Age of Expertise.* New York: Free Press, 1978.

Stauber, M. et al. "Psychosomatic Counseling of Couples Involved in An In Vitro Fertilization (IVF)-Embryo Transfer (ET) Program." *Experientia*, December 15, 1985, 41:1514–1515.

Steinfels, Margaret O'Brien. "In Vitro Fertilization: 'Ethically Acceptable' Research." *Hastings Center Report* (June 1979), 9:5–8.

Steptoe, P. C. and R. G. Edwards. "Reimplantation of a Human Embryo with Subsequent Tubal Pregnancy." *Obstetrical and Gynecological Survey* (October 1976), 31:750–752.

Stewart, Sandra and Greer Glazer. "Expectations and Coping of Women Undergoing In Vitro Fertilization." *Maternal-Child Nursing Journal* (Summer 1986), 15:103–113.

Sulzner, George T. "The Policy Process and the Uses of National Governmental Study Commissions." *Western Political Quarterly* (September 1971), 24:438–448.

Tauer, Carol A. "Personhood and Human Embryos and Fetuses." *Journal of Medicine and Philosophy* (August 1985), 10:253–266.

Tejeda, Rafael I. and William G. Karow. "Semantics Used in the Nomenclature of In Vitro Fertilization, or Let's All Be More Proper." *Journal of In Vitro Fertilization and Embryo Transfer* (1986), 3:341–342.

Templeton, A. A. et al. "What Potential Ovum Donors Think." *Lancet* (May 12, 1984), 1:8385:1081–1082.

Templeton, J. et al., "Activation of Nucleolar and Extranucleolar RNA Synthesis and Changes in the Ribosomal Content of Human Embryos Developing *In Vitro.*" *Journal of Reproduction and Fertility* (1986), 78:463–470.

Testart, Jacques, Bruno Lassalle, and Robert Forman, et al. "Factors Influencing the Success Rate of Human Embryo Freezing in an In Vitro Fertilization and Embryo Transfer Program." *Fertility and Sterility* (November 1987), 48:107–112.

Thomas, William, A., ed. *Scientists in the Legal System.* Ann Arbor, Mich.: Ann Arbor Science Publishers, 1974.

Tiefel, Hans O. "Human In Vitro Fertilization: A Conservative View." *Journal of the American Medical Association* (June 18, 1980), 247:3235–3242.

Tilton, Nan, Todd Tilton, and Gaylen Moore. *Making Miracles: In Vitro Fertilization.* Garden City, N.Y.: Doubleday, 1985.

Trounson, Alan. "Embryo Experimentation?" *Bioethics News* (July 1987), 6:n.p.

—— "Preservation of Human Eggs and Embryos." *Fertility and Sterility* (July 1986), 46:1–12.

Trounson, Alan and L. Mohr. "Human Pregnancy Following Cryopreservation, Thawing and Transfer of an Eight-Cell Embryo." *Nature* (1983), 350:707–709.

VLA Secretariat. "The Second Report of the Voluntary Licensing Authority for Human *In Vitro* Fertilisation and Embryology." London: The Voluntary Licensing Authority, April 1987.

——. "The Third Report of the Voluntary Licensing Authority for Human *In Vitro* Fertilisation and Embryology." London: The Voluntary Licensing Authority, April 1988.

Veeck, Lucinda L. *Atlas of the Human Oocyte and Early Conceptus. Baltimore: Williams and Wilkins, 1986.*

Venturatos-Lorio, Kathryn. "Alternative Means of Reproduction: Virgin Territory for Legislation." *Louisiana Law Review* (1984), 44:1641–1676.

Wadlington, Walter. "Artificial Conception: The Challenge for Family Law." *Virginia Law Review* (1983), 69:465–514.

Waller, Louis. "In Australia, The Debate Moves to Embryo Experimentation." *Hastings Center Report* (June 1987), 17:21S–24S.

Walters, LeRoy. "Ethics and New Reproductive Technologies: An International Review of Committee Statements." *Hastings Center Report* (June 1987), 17:3S–9S.

Walters, William A. W. and Peter Singer, eds. *Test-Tube Babies: A Guide to Moral Questions, Present Techniques and Future Possibilities.* Melbourne: Oxford University Press, 1982.

Warnock, Mary. *A Question of Life: The Warnock Report on Human Fertilisation and Embryology.* Oxford: Basil Blackwell, 1985.

Warren, Mary Anne. *Gendercide: The Implications of Sex Selection.* Totowa, N.J.: Rowman and Allanheld, 1985.

Watson, James D. "Moving Toward the Clonal Man—Is This What We Want?" *Congressional Record.* U.S. Senate, April 29, 1971, pp. 12751–12752.

Watt, J. L. et al. "Trisomy 1 in an Eight Cell Human Pre-Embryo." *Journal of Medical Genetics* (January 1987), 24:60–64.

West, John D. et al. "Sexing the Human Pre-Embryo by DNA and DNA In-Situ Hybridisation." *Lancet* (June 13, 1987), 1:8546:1345–1347.

"What You Should Know About Infertility." *Contemporary OB/GYN* (February 1980), 15:101–105.

Whitehead, Alfred North, *Symbolism: Its Meaning and Effect.* New York: Macmillan, 1927.

"Who Should Pay for Infertility?" *Hastings Center Report* (December 1987), 17:3–4.

Wikler, Norma Juliet. "Society's Response to the New Reproductive Technologies: The Feminist Perspectives." *Southern California Law Review* (July 1986), 59:1043–1057.

Wood, Carl et al. "Factors Influencing Pregnancy Rates Following In Vitro Fertilization and Embryo Transfer." *Fertility and Sterility* (February 1985), 43:245–250.

Wright, Germaine M. and James G. Zimmerly. "The Constitutional Right to Use In Vitro Fertilization." In Cyril H. Wecht, ed. *Legal Medicine,* pp. 239–255. Philadelphia: Sanders, 1982.

Zaner, Richard M. "A Criticism of Moral Conservatism's View of In Vitro Fertilization and Embryo Transfer." *Perspectives in Biology and Medicine* (Winter 1984), 27:200–212.

Ziporyn, Terra. " 'Artificial' Human Reproduction Poses Medical, Social Concerns." *Journal of the American Medical Association* (January 3, 1986), 255:13–15.

Index

Abortion, 22, 24, 76-77, 80-81, 89, 94, 97-98, 111, 113, 119, 129
Adoption, 20, 23-24, 94, 102-3
American College of Obstetricians and Gynecologists (ACOG), 87, 102, 121, 140
American Fertility Society (AFS), 85-90, 102, 140, 143; 1984 guidelines, 39-41, 43, 83, 87, 121; 1986 guidelines, 39, 87-89, 121
Andrews, Lori B., 163n38
Andrology, 27
Annas, George J., 165n64, 166n94
Arkansas insurance law, 102, 105
Artificial insemination by donor, 21, 94-96, 98, 117
Artificial womb, 1, 15, 132
Asexual reproduction, 132
Atwood, Margaret, 125-26
Australia, policy in, 92-93, 105-6, 134

Bible, procreation and, 123
Biomedical Ethics Board, 94
Bloom County, 119
Brown, Lesley, 17-18, 51, 76
Brown, Louise, 17-19, 81, 118, 120

Califano, Joseph, 78, 81
Callahan, Daniel, 103, 137

Cloning, 14, 15, 79, 92-93, 113
Compelling state interest test, 79, 93, 98, 115, 144
Consumption: circumspect, 6, 9, 48, 51, 64, 71-74, 110, 127, 138-39; uncircumspect, 6, 74, 142; principles of, 121-27, 142
Corea, Gena, 131-32, 171n40
Cost/benefit analysis, 88, 121, 124-27
Cranston, Alan, 102
Cross-species fertilization, 92-93

de Graaf, Reiner, 12
Del Zio, John and Doris, 16-18, 29, 56-57, 76, 145
Department of Health and Human Services (DHHS), 105
Department of Health, Education, and Welfare (DHEW), 77-78, 80-81, 121
Diesthystilbestrol (DES), 53, 102
Diffusion of innovations, 95
Distancing, 128-130
Doornbos v. Doornbos, 156n59
Dubler, Nancy, 134

Edwards, Robert, 13, 15, 17-18, 22, 29, 49, 76-77, 123, 128, 131-32
Egg: appearance, 149; donation, 88-89, 96, 105-6, 109, 117, 119-20, 125, 127; freezing, 40, 106-7, 143, 151

Eisenstadt v. Baird, 168n144
Ellis, Gary B., 94, 167n111
Embryo biopsy, 46, 101
Embryo freezing: 3, 5, 30-36, 45-48, 105-7, 115, 117, 130; advantages, 3, 30-31; consent forms, 32-33, 38-39, 41-44, 108; costs, 37, 72, 102, 105; decisions in programs, 36-45, 97, 141; emotional aspects of, 31, 33-36, 47; risks, 32; success rates, 32-33, 49, 72; time limitations, 36-38, 47
Embryo research: 42, 45-47, 79-82, 88; and IVF, 76-77, 81-82, 105-10, 122, 125; benefits, 106-10; creation of embryos for, 88, 106, 108-9; federal funding, 81; fourteen-day limit, 79, 93, 144; restrictions, 88-89, 93, 99, 101, 110, 139
Embryos: abnormal, 106, 108-9; appearance, 132, 150-51; as property, 40-43, 128, 130, 138; cross-generational transfer, 36, 118, 127-28; donation, 37-38, 48, 88, 96, 105, 119-20, 125, 127, 132; discarding, 43-45, 47, 93, 96, 106; nature of, 14, 40-42, 44, 79, 89, 96, 109, 122, 126-27, 130; patient bonding with, 40, 62-63; ranking of, 45, 109, 125, 151; relationship to couple, 42-43; rights of, 98
Embryo trafficking, 37, 97-98
Embryo transfer, 3, 63, 68, 151
Endocrinology, 27, 83
Endometriosis, 23, 70, 102
Ethics: definition, 120-21; IVF and, 18, 48-50, 55, 78-79, 104, 120-24, 129, 135, 141, 143
Ethics Advisory Board: creation, 77-78, 91, 121; disbanding, 81-82, 101, 105, 134; proposed reinstatement, 105; reaction to Report, 80-82; Report (1979), 79-82, 87, 139
Ethics committees, 30-31, 38-40, 77, 87, 121, 141
Etzioni, Amitai, 132
Experimentation and the unborn, 14-15, 122

Federal government and IVF: funding, 101, 105-10, 134, 144; history of, 76-

82, 89-91, 94-95; inaction and, 81, 90, 94, 111-12; national commission, 101, 112-16; responsibilities of, 112-16, 141-43
Feminism and IVF, 14, 125-26, 141
Fertilization, 27-28, 126, 132, 150-51
FINRRAGE, 125
Follicular monitoring, 59-60, 147
Food and Drug Administration, 94, 98
Frankenstein, 131-32

Gamete intrafallopian tube transfer (GIFT), 25, 86
Genetic defects, 5, 107-9, 116, 118-20, 143-44
Genetic engineering, 15, 79, 81, 108, 124, 129, 131
Glover, Jonathan, 128, 173n70
Gore, Albert, Jr., 90, 164-65n62, 168n146

Harris, Patricia, 81
Hawaii insurance law, 102
Hippocratic Oath, 46
Hodgkin, Paul, 155n44
Holmes, Oliver Wendell, 139
House Committee on Science and Technology, 90
Hulka, Jaroslav, 156n68
"Humster test," 22, 92-93
Huxley, Aldous, 14, 15, 131
Hysterosalpingogram, 20, 53

Idiopathic infertility, 19, 70
Illinois IVF law, 97, 98
Infertility: closure and, 35-36, 47, 64-67; history, 11-12, 19-24, 55-56, 119; isolation of, 52-54, 61, 126; loss and, 53-54; male, 20-21, 70, 92-93, 107; prevention of, 103-4; primary, 57; psychological aspects, 21-22, 52-58, 61, 63; secondary, 57; treatment, 22-24; veterans and, 102-3, 143; women and, 20-21
Infertility treatment, social importance of, 20-22, 103, 114, 143-44
Institutional Review Boards, 39, 80, 89, 91
Insurance and IVF, 5, 102-5, 110, 113-14
Intrauterine device (IUD), 1, 69
Intuition, 123-124

In vitro fertilization: access to, 101-5, 112, 115, 139; anxieties and, 14-15, 17, 130-35; artificiality of, 14, 18, 125, 129; as a political issue, 4, 81-82, 94, 100, 129; as dehumanizing, 2-3, 50, 126, 141; "basic," 5, 8, 90, 99, 101, 104, 112, 116, 121, 138, 145; benefits, 14, 23-24, 29, 78, 88-89, 108, 126, 138, 144; choices and, 5, 105, 114, 117-21, 127-28, 142; cost, 25, 78, 102-5, 110, 143; criticisms, 14, 80, 89, 104, 124-27; data collection, 79, 81, 86, 99-100, 116, 124, 141-42, 145; defects in offspring, 85; demystification of, 114, 134; emotional aspects, 14, 34, 47, 58-64, 66, 71, 141, 143; "expanded," 5-8, 36, 48, 51, 71, 74, 88, 90, 99-101, 104, 110, 112, 114, 116, 120-21, 124, 127-28, 130, 137-39, 144-45; experience of, 2, 58-64, 66, 140-41, 143, 147-51; history, 11-18, 56, 86, 128, 131, 137-38, 148; husband's role, 2-3, 60, 149; language of, 41, 44-47, 50, 128-30, 138, 144-45; legal aspects, 17-18, 41-42, 83-85, 140; public opinion, 18, 79, 114, 138; success rates, 24, 60-61, 68-72, 96, 140-43; symbols and, 11, 16-18, 22, 24-25, 40, 45-46, 50, 89, 104, 109, 114, 128-30, 138, 140, 144; values and, 6-9, 89, 127, 138-39
In vitro fertilization clinics, 24-30, 72, 83, 85, 99, 140, 143, 145
IVF Special Interest Group, 86

Jonas, Hans, 142
Jones, Howard W., Jr., 87, 168n133, 172n50
Journal of the American Medical Association, 81

Kass, Leon R., 18, 20, 47, 104, 124-25, 134
Klass, Perri, 73
Krause, Harry, 113, 163n38

Laparoscope, 22, 148
Laproscopy, 2, 26, 53, 60-61, 68, 148-49
Lejuene, Jerome, 171n43
Licensing, 93-95, 99, 115

Lindblom, Charles, 113
Louisiana: IVF law, 96, 98; surrogacy law, 97

McCartney, Cheryl, 58
Marketing of IVF, 26
Maryland insurance law, 102, 104, 140
Massachusetts: fetal research law: 96, 98; insurance law, 102, 105
Masturbation, 21, 125
Mazor, Miriam D., 156n57
Medical Research International, 100
Mendeloff, John, 162n22, 168n148
Menning, Barbara Eck, 22, 53
Metaphors, 45-46, 108, 110, 138, 145
Microwave ovens, 7-8
Miscarriage, 54, 60, 73, 107

National Conference of Commissioners on Uniform State Laws, 95
National Institutes of Health, 17, 77, 100, 113
National Right to Life Committee, 76
Nazism, 1, 80, 113
Nelkin, Dorothy, 134
Nurse coordinators, 26, 62, 66-67, 141

Office of Technology Assessment, 94, 103, 142
"Orphaned" embryos, 41, 84
Orwell, George, 117, 138
Ovum transfer, 45, 56, 88, 117

Paternalism, 55, 64, 72
Patients: autonomy, 51, 64, 70-71; decision making, 46-47, 67-71; desperation, 5, 23-24, 29, 47, 56-58, 129-30, 138; over age forty, 24, 49, 70, 73; resolutions from IVF, 47, 64-67; responsibilities and, 71-74, 85, 99, 129, 134, 141, 143; vulnerability, 46, 51-58, 72, 140-41
Pellegrino, Edmund, 143
Pelvic inflammatory disease, 23
Pennsylvania IVF law, 97, 100
Physicians: as gatekeepers, 25, 40, 45, 47, 50; responsibilities of, 43, 45-50, 66-67, 90, 128, 140-43; regulation of IVF, 82-92

Pope Pius XII, 122
Pregnancies: chemical, 60-61, 69, 151; clinical, 61, 69, 86, 151; ectopic, 23, 54-55, 69, 128
Private sector regulation: advantages, 82-90, 99-100, 114, 140-42; incentives, 83-86; problems, 87, 90, 140-141; types, 86-90, 98-100, 115
Procreation, freedom of, 75, 79, 88-90, 96, 105, 111-12, 114-16
Proximity and degree test, 93
Public policy: affirmative, 91, 100-11, 138, 144; incremental model of, 75, 95, 99-100, 102, 110, 112-13, 115, 137-42, 145; prohibitions, 91-93; regulations, 91-100, 115; see also Federal government and IVF; State governments

Quindlen, Anna, 127

Ramsey, Paul, 15, 76, 91, 103, 122, 125
Resolve, Inc., 22
Rifkin, Jeremy, 134, 173n71
Robertson, John A., 167n127-128, 168nn134, 141
Roe v. Wade, 22, 24, 97, 161n6, 168n145

Schroeder, Patricia, 102
Scientists: IVF and, 82, 87-89, 92-93, 107; public mistrust of, 115-16, 131-32, 139
Shettles, Landrum, 12, 16-18, 29, 49, 76
Skinner v. Oklahoma, 168n143
Slippery slope, 3, 110, 115, 129, 137-38
Society of Assisted Reproductive Technology (SART), 86, 99
Soupart, Pierre, 76-80, 89, 106
Sperm, quality of, 149-150

Standing Review and Advisory Committee, 106
State governments: fetal research statutes, 77, 96-97, 101; laboratories for policy, 95-96, 144; modeling among, 95, 99-100, 102, 113; role in IVF, 75, 95-100, 102-5, 113-14, 144
Statutory Licensing Authority, 93
Steptoe, Patrick, 13, 17-18, 22, 77, 128
Stern, Elizabeth and William, 118
Strindberg, August, 133
Supreme Court, U.S., 88, 98, 111, 114, 122
Surrogate motherhood: 88, 94, 118-20, 124, 127; as option, 8, 56, 58; Baby M case, 84, 118-19, 127; complications, 84, 118; state laws, 95-96

Technological imperative, 6, 92, 134, 138
"Test-tube babies," 1, 2, 5, 11, 14-15, 17-18, 114, 117, 125, 129-31, 138
Texas insurance law, 102, 105
Tubal infertility, 22-23, 69-70, 102, 116
Tubal ligation, 23, 57-58, 120
Tubal surgery, 23

Ultrasonography, 147, 149, 151

van Buren, Abigail, 117-18, 120
Vande Wiele, Raymond, 16-17
Vatican, 122
Voluntary Licensing Authority (VLA), 93

Warnock Report, 91, 93, 123
Watson, James, 76
Whitehead, Alfred North, 7, 24, 153n1
Whitehead, Mary Beth, 118

Zola, Irving, 172n57